YOGA FOR DUMMIES®

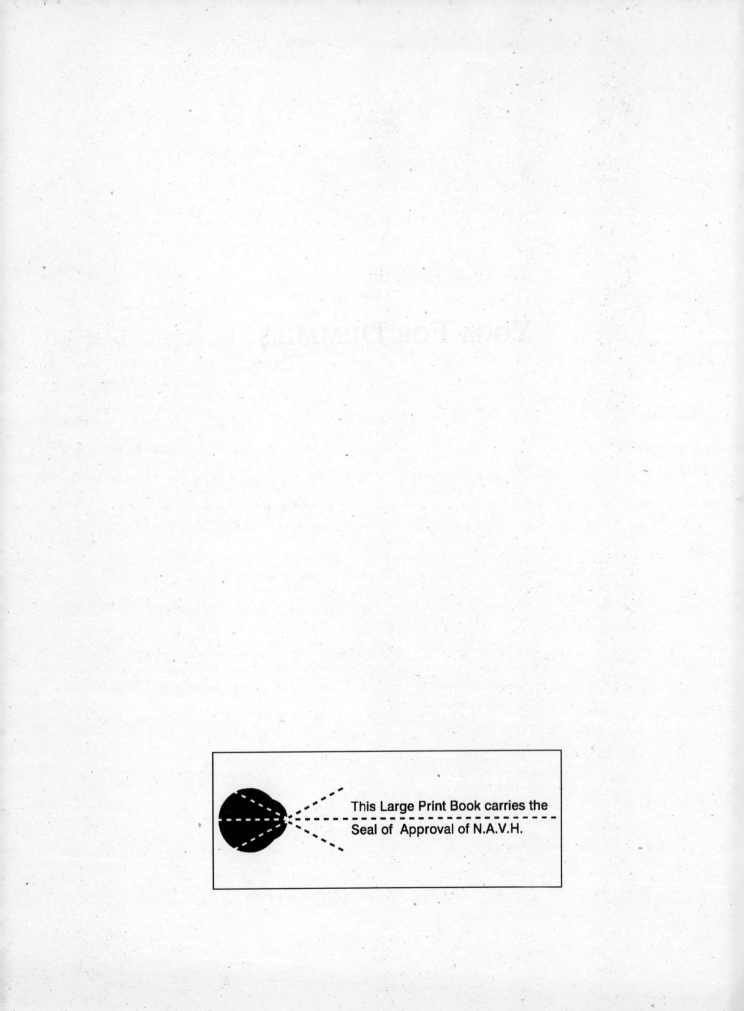

This Large Print Book carries the
Seal of Approval of N.A.V.H.

YOGA FOR DUMMIES®

2nd Edition

GEORG FEUERSTEIN, PhD
AND LARRY PAYNE, PhD

THORNDIKE PRESS
A part of Gale, Cengage Learning

 GALE
CENGAGE Learning™

Detroit • New York • San Francisco • New Haven, Conn • Waterville, Maine • London

GALE
CENGAGE Learning

LIBRARY OF CONGRESS CATALOGING-IN-PUBLICATION DATA

Feuerstein, Georg.
  Yoga for dummies / by Georg Feuerstein and Larry Payne. -- Large print ed.
    p. cm.
  ISBN-13: 978-1-4104-2831-8 (hardcover)
  ISBN-10: 1-4104-2831-1 (hardcover)
  1. Hatha yoga. 2. Large type books. I. Payne, Larry. II. Title.
RA781.7.F48 2010
613.7'046--dc22
                                                    2010013908

Published in 2010 in arrangement with John Wiley & Sons, Inc.

Printed in the United States of America
1 2 3 4 5 6 7 14 13 12 11 10

AUG   2010

Dedication

. . . .

From Larry: My contribution to this book is dedicated to the love of my life Merry Aronson, my beloved family, Dolly, Harry in heaven, Chris, Harold, Susan, Lisa, Natale, Maria, and my students who have been my greatest teachers.

About the Authors

Georg Feuerstein, PhD, has been studying and practicing Yoga since his early teens and is a practitioner of Buddhist Yoga. He is internationally respected for his contribution to Yoga research and the history of consciousness and has been featured in many national magazines both in the United States and abroad. He has authored over 40 books, including *The Yoga Tradition, The Shambhala Encyclopedia of Yoga,* and *Yoga Morality,* which have been translated into eight languages. Since his retirement in 2004, he has designed and tutored several distance-learning courses on Yoga philosophy for Traditional Yoga Studies, a Canadian company founded and directed by his wife, Brenda (see www.traditionalyogastudies.com).

Larry Payne, PhD, is an internationally prominent Yoga teacher, author, workshop leader, and pioneer in the field of Yoga therapy since 1980. He discovered Yoga when he was challenged by his own serious back problems and injuries from numerous competitive sports played in his youth.

Larry is co-founder of the Yoga curriculum at the UCLA School of Medicine. He was named "One of America's most respected Yoga teachers" by the *Los Angeles Times,* and was selected as a leading Yoga expert by Dr. Mehmet Oz, *Reader's Digest,* Web-MD, Rodale Press, and the *Yoga Journal.*

In Los Angeles, Larry is founding director of the Yoga Therapy Rx and Prime of Life Yoga certification programs at Loyola Marymount University and has a thriving private practice in Yoga therapy as a back specialist. He is coauthor of five books and is featured in the DVD series *Yoga Therapy Rx* and *Prime of Life Yoga.* His Web site is www. samata.com.

Author's Acknowledgments

From Georg: I would like to cordially thank Larry for graciously shouldering the main burden of preparing this new edition for the press. My thanks also go to the *For Dummies* staff for their essential behind-the-scenes work done.

From Larry: Unless you are truly gifted like my coauthor Georg, writing a book takes a village, and I have many people to thank in mine. Merry of MerryMedia first encouraged me to do this revision. Sri TKV Desikachar and his family have inspired my Yoga path since 1980. My editor, Deborah Myers, was simply grand. My council of advisors is always there for me: Prof. Zhuo-Yi Qiu, OMD; David Allen, MD; Richard Usatine, MD; Rick Morris, DC; Richard Miller, PhD; Art Brownstein, MD; Mike Sinel, MD; Prof. Sasi Velupillai, Steve Ostrow, JD; and my personal assistant, Jenna Entwistle.

Michael Lewis at Wiley initiated this revision project, and his patience and persistence made it happen. Thanks also go to Carol Susan Roth, our book agent, and our editorial team at Wiley, led by Chrissy Guthrie and Megan Knoll who are both talented and compassionate.

I am very grateful to our photographer, Adam Latham, and

our 21 models starring Jeffrey Aronson, Michael Aronson, Deborah Barry, Holly Beaty, Anna Brown, Chauncey Dennis, Lili Foster, Mia Foster, Terra Gold, Eden Goldman, Anna Inferrera, Marvin Jordana, Chris Joseph, the Ketterhagen family: Kourtney, Luke, Mangala, and Prakash, Dolly Payne, Tony Ransdell, Heidi Rayden, and Vivian Richman.

Publisher's Acknowledgments

We're proud of this book; please send us your comments at http://dummies.custhelp.com. For other comments, please contact our Customer Care Department within the U.S. at 877-762-2974, outside the U.S. at 317-572-3993, or fax 317-572-4002.

Some of the people who helped bring this book to market include the following:

Acquisitions, Editorial, and Media Development

Senior Project Editor: Christina Guthrie
(Previous Edition: Jennifer Ehrlich)
Acquisitions Editor: Michael Lewis
Copy Editor: Megan Knoll
Assistant Editor: Erin Calligan Mooney
Editorial Program Coordinator: Joe Niesen
Technical Editor: Jen Xanders
Editorial Manager: Christine Meloy Beck
Editorial Assistant: Jennette ElNaggar
Art Coordinator: Alicia B. South
Cartoons: Rich Tennant (www.the5thwave.com)

Composition Services for Original Edition

Project Coordinator: Katherine Crocker
Layout and Graphics: Carl Byers, Joyce Haughey, Brent Savage, Christine Williams
Proofreaders: John Greenough, Betty Kish
Indexer: Cheryl Duksta
Special Art: Interior photos by Adam Latham

Publishing and Editorial for Consumer Dummies

Diane Graves Steele, Vice President and Publisher, Consumer Dummies
Kristin Ferguson-Wagstaffe, Product Development Director, Consumer Dummies
Ensley Eikenburg, Associate Publisher, Travel
Kelly Regan, Editorial Director, Travel

Publishing for Technology Dummies

Andy Cummings, Vice President and Publisher, Dummies Technology/General User

Composition Services

Debbie Stailey, Director of Composition Services

Contents at a Glance

14

Table of Contents

19

Introduction

More than 15 million Americans practice Yoga of one kind or another, and many more millions of Yoga practitioners live in other parts of the world. Yoga isn't a fad. It has been around in the West for well over a hundred years and has a history of approximately five millennia. It's clearly here to stay, so don't worry that you're investing yourself in some flash-in-the-pan phenomenon that will disappear six months from now.

Yoga may be 5,000 years old, but the modern Yoga boom didn't start until the 1960s, largely thanks to Richard Hittleman's extraordinarily successful TV series *Yoga for Health*. This show was followed in the 1970s by Lilias Folan's TV series *Lilias, Yoga and You.* This era also brought the rise of Transcendental Meditation (TM) — a form of Yoga — largely because of the Beatles' interest in it. TM attracted hundreds of thousands who were in search of stress reduction and a more meaningful life.

Yoga has brought health and peace of mind to millions of people, and it can do the same for you. We challenge you to explore Yoga in depth, with *Yoga For Dummies,* 2nd Edition, as your guide. The yogic postures are an excellent starting point, but they're merely the outermost shell of a multilayered tradition. At its core, Yoga is a timeless answer for those who quest for a deeper meaning in life and for that elusive treasure called abiding peacefulness.

About This Book

Perhaps *Yoga For Dummies,* 2nd Edition, is the first book on Yoga you've ever held in your hands. In this case, we can confidently say that you're starting at the right place. More likely, however, you have leafed through quite a few other books (there is definitely no shortage of publications dealing with Yoga exercises). Not all of those publications are either sound or helpful. Why, then, should you take this book seriously? We have a two-part answer for you.

First, the information you find in *Yoga For Dummies,* 2nd Edition, is based on our extensive study and practice of Yoga. Between us, we have 75 years of experience with Yoga. One author (Georg) is internationally recognized as a leading expert on the Yoga tradition and has authored many seminal works on it (some of which we list in the appendix) and has created a teacher training manual on Yoga philosophy used by many Yoga teachers in seven countries. The other author (Larry) directs a university-based Yoga therapy training program for Yoga teachers at Loyola Marymount University; has a thriving practice as a Yoga teacher and Yoga therapist in Los Angeles, where he teaches and responds to his clients' specific health challenges, notably back problems; and has produced a popular series of Yoga DVDs (also listed in the appendix). In this book, we merge our respective areas of expertise to create a reliable and user-friendly introductory book that can also serve you as a beginner's reference work on an ongoing basis.

Second, we're both dedicated to motivating you to practice this system, which we have seen work minor and major miracles. We have committed our lives to making Yoga available to anyone who cares about the health and wholeness of the body and mind. In short (and without feeling self-important), we can say that you're in the best of hands.

This book guides you slowly, step by step, into the treasure house of Yoga. And it's a fabulous treasure house! You find out how to strengthen your mind and enlist it to unlock your body's extraordinary potential. A sound body requires a sound mind, and we show you how to improve or regain the health and wholeness of both.

Whether you're interested in becoming more flexible, fitter, less stressed out, or more peaceful and joyful, this book contains all the good counsel and practical exercises to start you in the right direction.

Above all, we have endeavored to make this book relevant to busy people like you. And if, after reading this guide, you become more serious about studying and practicing Yoga, consider taking a Yoga class with a qualified instructor. This book is a great guide, but nothing compares to hands-on teaching.

Conventions Used in This Book

To help you work your way through this book, we've set up a few conventions:

- **Boldfaced** text emphasizes keywords in bulleted lists and identifies steps to take in numbered lists.

- New terms are *italicized* and followed closely by a definition.

- URLs appear in monofont.

- In English, you customarily write *yoga* in lower-case letters. However, throughout this book, we write the word with an initial capital letter — *Yoga* — to emphasize that Yoga is a self-contained system or tradition, like Zen, Hinduism, or Buddhism. The adjective of Yoga is *yogic,* which you encounter frequently in this book.

- A person who's dedicated to balancing mind and body through Yoga is traditionally called a *yogi* (if male) or a *yogini* (if female), and we use both terms. Alternatively, we also use the English term Yoga practitioner.

- Although we give you some basic info on all branches of Yoga, the focus of this book is on Hatha (pronounced *haht-ha*) Yoga, which is the branch that works primarily with the body through postures, breathing exercises, and other similar techniques.

- We use the words *pose* and *posture* interchangeably, although we use *posture* in the names of specific postures.

A final note: For your safety, be sure to read all the instructions when getting ready to practice the exercises. Don't just glance at the illustrations and think you can leap right in. Although the illustrations are very helpful tools, they don't give you the whole story needed to practice safe and effective Yoga.

What You're Not to Read

We must admit that we hope you read every word in this

book at some point in your yogic journey. We also confess that we include a few tidbits just to get your mind going and make you think. We mark this text with the Technical Stuff icon or format it as a *sidebar* (shaded gray box). These tidbits are interesting and important in their own right, but they're not essential to your practice of the various postures. Feel free to skip 'em, but plan to go back and read them at some point. You'll be glad you did!

Foolish Assumptions

We're not here to judge, but we have made some general assumptions about you, the reader. First, we assume that you're interested in reaping some benefits from practicing Yoga. Second, we assume that you don't have much (if any) experience with Yoga. Finally, we assume that you're curious and willing to find out more. That's it. Nothing fancy. If you fall into any of these categories, *Yoga For Dummies,* 2nd Edition, is for you!

How This Book Is Organized

This book is organized according to the characteristic design of all *For Dummies* books. It answers all the important questions you need to know for a successful practice of Yoga.

Yoga For Dummies is conveniently divided into five parts. Here is what you can expect to encounter in them:

Part I: Off to a Good Start with Yoga

This opening part sets the stage for the discussions and practices that follow and covers some of the fundamentals you need to know before beginning with the postures. In Chapter 1, we explain what Yoga is and clear up some widespread misunderstandings about it. We also introduce the five basic approaches to and twelve principal branches of Yoga and review how these relate to your health and happiness. In Chapter 2, we provide you with down-to-earth practical advice on getting started with your own Yoga practice, showing you how you can make it both safe and effective. In particular, we answer all your questions about participating in a class or practicing on your own. Chapter 3 covers everything you need to do to prepare for a Yoga session, including cultivating the right state of mind. Chapter 4 introduces the art of relaxation, which is fundamental to a successful Yoga practice. In Chapter 5, we explain the importance of correct breathing both during the execution of the Yoga postures and as a discipline in its own right.

Part II: Postures for Health Maintenance and Restoration

In the second part, we jump straight into the Yoga postures. In Chapters 6 through 13, you successively discover sitting postures, standing postures, balancing exercises, special practices for your abdominals, inversions, bends, and twists, as well as the popular dynamic movement called the Sun Salutation. In Chapter 14, we guide you through a short, time-tested routine designed for beginners.

Part III: Creative Yoga

Chapter 15 helps you spice it up and gives you the key formula to design well-rounded routines of varying lengths, as well as guidelines to ensure your practice is safe as well as enjoyable. In Chapters 16, 17, and 18, we delve into Yoga for different ages and stages — pregnancy through the senior years — and provide guidelines, suggest postures, and outline routines so that all potential yogis and yoginis can find their niches. Chapter 19 discusses the use of props and reviews simple props, such as walls, chairs, straps, and blocks, to facilitate your posture practice.

Part IV: Yoga as a Lifestyle

When you adopt Yoga as a lifestyle, your practice extends over the entire day. In this part, we explain how to make this shift and why this choice makes sense. As we show in Chapter 20, Yoga has much to say about positive mental attitudes toward work, leisure, diet, family, and other people. In Chapter 21, we introduce you to the art of meditation. If the postures are Yoga's backbone, meditation is its heart. Regular meditation puts you in touch with the joy and peace that is your mind's natural condition. Chapter 22 looks at using Yoga therapeutically to deal with common aches and pains and illustrates safe postures to relieve back pain. It also offers a five-step program to help you prevent chronic back pain so that you can continue, not curtail, your lifestyle. We also discuss how to find a good Yoga therapist.

Part V: The Part of Tens

All *For Dummies* books have a Part of Tens section, and this one is no different. Here we give you top-ten lists that provide you with useful and practical information. In Chapter 23, we let you in on important hints for a successful and enjoyable Yoga practice with a focus on relaxation, and Chapter 24 tells you the best places to visit in the

United States and Canada if you're interested in practicing Yoga with a competent teacher and/or in a group setting. Finally, in Chapter 25, we list ten good reasons for practicing Yoga.

We encourage you to explore Yoga further, so the appendix at the end of the book gives you the necessary resources to do just that. We cover prominent organizations and list some of the best Web sites, books, DVDs, audiotapes, and videos on the various aspects of Yoga.

Icons Used in This Book

Throughout this book, you may notice little pictures in the margins. You can use these icons as helpful pointers to information you don't want to forget (or, in some cases, don't want to read at all).

Following is the list of icons used in this book:

This icon points you toward helpful information that can make your yogic journey a little smoother.

Be sure to check out the information marked by this icon; it points out potential dangers you want to avoid.

This icon marks nerdy technical stuff that's interesting to know but probably not necessary to your understanding of Yoga. But you may be able to impress your friends at your next dinner party.

The paragraphs sitting next to this baby are pretty noteworthy. You may want to jot them down somewhere or circle them in the book for later reference.

Where to Go from Here

We've designed *Yoga For Dummies,* 2nd Edition, to be both an introduction and a beginner's reference work. You can read the chapters one after the other and practice along with us, or you can dip into the book here and there, reading up on the things that currently interest you, such as how to find the right kind of style or Yoga class for your needs, or what helpful props you can use to make your practice easier.

If you're a newcomer to Yoga, we recommend that you spend some time with the table of contents. You may even want to leaf through the book to get a general sense of how we have structured and approached the material.

If you aren't new to Yoga and simply want a refresher course, you can also use this book as a reliable guide in answering your questions. Just flip to the index to locate the information you need or check out the appendix, which refers you to a variety of sources of information on specific topics relating to Yoga. What are you waiting for? Dig in!

Part I

Off to a Good Start with Yoga

The 5th Wave   By Rich Tennant

"Okay, you've got the breathing down, but wouldn't you be more comfortable in a different workout suit?"

In this part . . .

Yoga is very comprehensive and includes a great variety of approaches. Before you go off hiking in the countryside, you need to take a quick look at the map or risk getting lost. Likewise, before you start experimenting with Yoga, you want to know what it is and how it works. That's how you can ensure that your practice of Yoga is both enjoyable and safe.

In this first part, we give you a road map that allows you to take the first steps in what will be an exciting and rewarding journey of discovery. We cover some of the fundamentals that can serve you well as you embark upon your practice of Yoga postures: guidelines for a safe practice, conscious breathing and relaxation techniques, and coordination of breath and movement.

Chapter 1

Yoga 101: What You Need to Know

Three or four decades ago, some people still occasionally confused *Yoga* with *yogurt*. Today, Yoga is a household word. The fact that just about everyone has heard the word *Yoga,* however, doesn't mean they know exactly what it means. Many misconceptions still exist, even among those who practice Yoga, so in this chapter, we clear up the confusion and explain what Yoga really is and how it relates to your health and happiness. We also help you see that Yoga, with its many different branches and approaches, really does offer something for everyone.

Whatever your age, weight, flexibility, or beliefs may be, you can practice and benefit from some version of Yoga.

41

Although Yoga originated in India, it's for all of humanity.

Understanding the True
Character of Yoga

Whenever you hear that Yoga is *just* this or *just* that, your
nonsense alert should kick into action. Yoga is too comprehensive to reduce to any one thing — it's like a skyscraper
with many floors and numerous rooms at each level. Yoga
isn't just gymnastics, fitness training, huffing and puffing,
or a way to control your weight. It's not just stress reduction, meditation, or some spiritual tradition from India.

Yoga is all these things and a great deal more. (You'd
expect as much from a tradition that's been around for
5,000 years.) Yoga includes physical exercises that look like
gymnastics and have even been incorporated into Western
gymnastics. These postural exercises help you become or
stay fit and trim, control your weight, and reduce your
stress level. Yoga also offers a whole range of meditation
practices, including breathing techniques that exercise your
lungs and calm your nervous system or charge your brain
and the rest of your body with delicious energy.

You can also use Yoga as an efficient system of health care
that has proven its usefulness in both restoring and maintaining health. Yoga continues to gain acceptance within
the medical establishment; more and more physicians are
recommending Yoga to their patients not only for stress reduction but also as a safe and sane method of exercise and
physical therapy (notably, for the back and knees).

But Yoga is more than even a system of preventative or
restorative health care. Yoga looks at health from a broad,

holistic perspective that's only now being rediscovered by avant-garde medicine. This perspective appreciates the enormous influence of the mind — your psychological attitudes — on physical health.

Finding unity

The word *Yoga* comes from the ancient Sanskrit language spoken by the traditional religious elite of India, the *Brahmins*. Yoga means "union" or "integration" and also "discipline," so the system of Yoga is called a *unitive* or *integrating discipline*. Yoga seeks unity at various levels. First, it seeks to unite body and mind, which people all too often separate. Some people are chronically "out of the body." They can't feel their feet or the ground beneath them, as if they hover like ghosts just above their bodies. They're unable to cope with the ordinary pressures of daily life and collapse under stress, and they're often confused and don't understand their own emotions. They're afraid of life and easily emotionally hurt.

Yoga also seeks to unite the rational mind and the emotions. People frequently bottle up their emotions and don't express their real feelings, choosing instead to rationalize these feelings away. Chronic avoidance can become a serious health hazard; if people aren't aware that they're suppressing feelings such as anger, the anger consumes them from the inside out.

Here's how Yoga can help you with your personal growth:

✔ **It can put you in touch with your real feelings and balance your emotional life.**

✔ **It can help you understand and accept yourself and feel comfortable with who you are.** You don't have to "fake it" or reduce your life to constant role-playing.

✔ **It helps you become more able to empathize and communicate with others.**

Yoga is a powerful means of psychological integration. It makes you aware that you're part of a larger whole, not merely an island unto yourself. Humans can't thrive in isolation. Even the most independent individual is greatly indebted to others. After your mind and body are happily reunited, this union with others comes about naturally. The moral principles of Yoga are all-embracing, encouraging you to seek kinship with everyone and everything. We say more about this topic in Chapter 20.

Finding yourself: Are you a yogi (or yogini)?

Someone who's practicing the discipline of balancing mind and body through Yoga is traditionally called a *yogi* (if male) or a *yogini* (if female). In this book, we use both terms at random. Alternatively, we also use the English term *Yoga practitioner*. In our book, practicing Yoga postures is a step in the right direction but doesn't make a person a *yogi* or *yogini*. For that, you'd have to embrace Yoga as a self-transforming spiritual discipline. A yogi or yogini who has really mastered Yoga is called an *adept*. If such an adept also teaches (and not all of them do), he or she is traditionally called a *guru*. The Sanskrit word *guru* means literally "weighty one." According to traditional esoteric sources, the syllable *gu* signifies spiritual darkness and *ru* signifies the act of removing. Thus a guru is a teacher who leads the student from darkness to light.

Very few Westerners have achieved complete mastery of Yoga, mainly because Yoga is still a relatively young movement in the West. So please be careful about those who claim to be enlightened or to have been given the title of guru! However, at the level at which Yoga is generally taught outside its Indian homeland, many competent Yoga teachers or instructors can lend a helping hand to beginners. In this book, we hope to do just that for you.

Considering Your Options: The Eight Main Branches of Yoga

When you take a bird's-eye view of the Yoga tradition, you see a dozen major strands of development, each with its own subdivisions. Picture Yoga as a giant tree with eight branches; each branch has its own unique character, but each is also part of the same tree. With so many different paths, you're sure to find one that's right for your personality, lifestyle, and goals. In this book we focus on Hatha Yoga, the most popular branch of Yoga, but we avoid the common mistake of reducing it to mere physical fitness training. Thus, we also talk about meditation and the spiritual aspects of Yoga.

Here are the seven principal branches of Yoga, arranged alphabetically:

- **Bhakti** *(bhuk-tee)* **Yoga:** The Yoga of devotion

- **Hatha** *(haht-ha)* **Yoga:** The Yoga of physical discipline

- **Jnana** *(gyah-nah)* **Yoga:** The Yoga of wisdom

- **Karma** *(kahr-mah)* **Yoga:** The Yoga of self-transcending action

- **Mantra** *(mahn-trah)* **Yoga:** The Yoga of potent sound

- **Raja** (rah-jah) **Yoga:** The Royal Yoga
- **Tantra** (tahn-trah) **Yoga (including Laya Yoga and Kundalini Yoga):** The Yoga of continuity

To this list we must add as a branch of its own *Guru (goo-roo) Yoga,* the Yoga of dedication to a Yoga master.

The seven branches and Guru Yoga are described in the following sections.

Bhakti Yoga: The Yoga of devotion

Bhakti Yoga practitioners believe that a supreme being (the Divine) transcends their lives, and they feel moved to connect or even completely merge with that supreme being through acts of devotion. Bhakti Yoga includes such practices as making flower offerings, singing hymns of praise, and thinking about the Divine.

Feeling enlightened

To get a sense of the nature of enlightenment, sit in a warm room as still as possible, with your hands in your lap. Now sense your skin all over; it's your body's boundary separating you from the air surrounding you. As you become more aware of your body's sensations, pay special attention to the connection between your skin and the air. After a while, you realize that no sharp boundary really exists between your skin and the outside air. In your imagination, you can extend yourself further and further beyond your skin into the surrounding space. Where do you end, and where does the space begin? This experience can give you a sense of the all-comprising expansiveness of enlightenment, which knows no boundaries.

Hatha Yoga: The Yoga of physical discipline

All branches of Yoga seek to achieve the same final goal, enlightenment (see Chapter 21), but Hatha Yoga approaches this goal through the body rather than through the mind or the emotions. Hatha Yoga practitioners believe that unless they properly purify and prepare their bodies, the higher stages of meditation and beyond are virtually impossible to achieve — such an attempt would be like trying to climb Mt. Everest without the necessary gear. We focus on this particular branch of Yoga in this book.

Hatha Yoga is very much more than posture practice, which is so popular today. Like every form of authentic Yoga, it's a *spiritual* path.

Jnana Yoga: The Yoga of wisdom

Jnana Yoga teaches the ideal of *nondualism* — that reality is singular, and your perception of countless distinct phenomena is a basic misconception. What about the chair or sofa that you're sitting on? Isn't that real? What about the light that strikes your retina? Isn't that real? Jnana Yoga masters answer these questions by saying that all these things are real at your present level of consciousness, but they aren't ultimately real as separate or distinct things. Upon enlightenment, everything melts into one, and you become one with the immortal spirit.

Karma Yoga: The Yoga of self-transcending action

Karma Yoga's most important principle is to act unselfishly, without attachment, and with integrity. Karma Yoga practitioners believe that all actions, whether bodily, vocal,

Good karma, bad karma, no karma

The Sanskrit term *karma* literally means "action." It stands for activity in general but also for the "invisible action" of destiny. According to Yoga, every action of body, speech, and mind produces visible and also hidden consequences. Sometimes the hidden consequences — destiny — are far more significant than the obvious repercussions. Don't think of karma as blind destiny. You're always free to make choices. The purpose of Karma Yoga is to regulate how you act in the world so that you cease to be bound by karma. The practitioners of all types of Yoga seek to not only prevent bad (black) karma but also go beyond good (white) karma to no karma at all.

or mental, have far-reaching consequences for which they must assume full responsibility.

Mantra Yoga: The Yoga of potent sound

Mantra Yoga makes use of sound to harmonize the body and focus the mind. It works with *mantras,* which can be a syllable, word, or phrase. Traditionally, practitioners receive a mantra from their teacher in the context of a formal initiation. They're asked to repeat it as often as possible and to keep it secret. Many Western teachers feel that initiation isn't necessary and that any sound works. You can even pick a word from the dictionary, such as *love, peace,* or *happiness,* but from a traditional perspective, such words are, strictly speaking, *not mantras.*

Raja Yoga: The Royal Yoga

Raja Yoga means literally "Royal Yoga" and is also known as *Classical Yoga*. When you mingle with Yoga students long enough, you can expect to hear them refer to the eightfold path laid down in the *Yoga-Sutra* of Patanjali, the standard work of Raja Yoga. Another name for this yogic tradition is *Ashtanga Yoga* (pronounced *ahsh-tahng-gah*), the "eight-limbed Yoga" — from *ashta* ("eight") and *anga* ("limb"). (Don't confuse this tradition with the Yoga style known as Ashtanga Yoga, which we discuss in "Getting The Scoop on the Prominent Styles of Hatha Yoga" later in this chapter.) The eight limbs of the prominent traditional approach, designed to lead to enlightenment or liberation, are as follows:

- **Yama (yah-mah):** Moral discipline, consisting of the practices of nonharming, truthfulness, nonstealing, chastity, and greedlessness (for an explanation of these five virtues, head to Chapter 20).

- **Niyama (nee-yah-mah):** Self-restraint, consisting of the five practices of purity, contentment, austerity, self-study, and devotion to a higher principle.

- **Asana (ah-sah-nah):** Posture, which serves two basic purposes: meditation and health.

- **Pranayama (prah-nah-yah-mah):** Breath control, which raises and balances your mental energy, thus boosting your health and mental concentration.

- **Pratyahara (prah-tyah-hah-rah):** Sensory inhibition, which internalizes your consciousness to prepare your mind for the various stages of meditation.

- **Dharana (dhah-rah-nah):** Concentration, or extended mental focusing, which is fundamental to yogic meditation.

- **Dhyana (dhee-yah-nah):** Meditation, the principal practice of higher Yoga (this practice and the next are explained in Chapter 21).

✔ **Samadhi (sah-mah-dhee):** Ecstasy, or the experience in which you become inwardly one with the object of your contemplation. This state is surpassed by actual enlightenment, or spiritual liberation.

Tantra Yoga: The Yoga of continuity

Tantra Yoga is the most complex and most widely misunderstood branch of Yoga. In the West and in India, Tantra

The sacred syllable *om*

The best known traditional mantra, used by Hindus and Buddhists alike, is the sacred syllable *om* (pronounced *ommm,* with a long *o* sound). It's the symbol of the absolute reality — the Self or spirit. It's composed of the letters *a, u,* and *m* and the nasal humming of the letter *m. A* corresponds to the waking state, *u* to the dream state, and *m* to the state of deep sleep; the nasal humming sound represents the ultimate reality. We introduce several other traditional mantras in Chapter 21 in our coverage of meditation.

Yoga is often confused with "spiritualized" sex; although sexual rituals are used in some (so-called left-hand) schools of Tantra Yoga, they aren't a regular practice in the majority of (so-called right-hand) schools. Tantra Yoga is actually a strict spiritual discipline involving fairly complex rituals and detailed visualizations of deities. These deities are either visions of the divine or the equivalent of Christianity's angels and are invoked to aid the yogic process of contemplation.

Another common name for Tantra Yoga is Kundalini Yoga (pronounced *koon-dah-lee-nee*). The latter name, which means "she who is coiled," hints at the secret "serpent power" that Tantra Yoga seeks to activate: the latent spiritual energy stored in the human body. If you're curious about this aspect of Yoga, you may want to read the autobiographical account by Gopi Krishna (see the appendix) or my (Georg's) *Tantra: The Path of Ecstasy* (Shambhala). **Note:** Kundalini Yoga is also the name of a Hatha Yoga style; we discuss it in "Getting The Scoop on the Prominent Styles of Hatha Yoga" later in the chapter.

Guru Yoga: The Yoga of dedication to a master

In Guru Yoga, your teacher is the main focus of spiritual practice. Such a teacher is expected to be enlightened or at least close to being enlightened (see Chapter 21 for more about enlightenment). In Guru Yoga, you honor and meditate on your guru until you merge with him or her. Because the guru is thought to already be one with the ultimate reality, this merger duplicates his or her spiritual realization in you.

But, please, don't merge too readily! This Yoga is relatively rare in the West, so approach it with great caution to avoid possible exploitation.

Getting The Scoop on the Prominent Styles of Hatha Yoga

In its voyage to modernity, Yoga has undergone many transformations. One of them was Hatha Yoga, which emerged around 1100 AD. The most significant adaptations, however, were made during the past several decades, particularly to serve the needs or wants of Western students. Of the many styles of Hatha Yoga available today, the following are the best known:

- **Iyengar Yoga,** which is the most widely recognized approach to Hatha Yoga, was created by B. K. S. Iyengar, the brother in-law of the famous T.S. Krishnamacharya (1888–1989) and uncle of T.K.V. Desikachar. This style is characterized by precision performance and the aid of numerous props. Iyengar has trained thousands of teachers, many of whom are in the United States. His Ramamani Iyengar Memorial Yoga Institute, founded in 1974 and dedicated to his late wife Ramamani, is located in Pune, India.

- **Viniyoga** (pronounced *vee-nee yoh-gah*) is the approach first developed by Shri Krishnamacharya and continued with his son T.K.V. Desikachar. The emphasis is on the breath and practicing Yoga according to your individual needs and capacities. In the United States, Viniyoga is now associated with Gary Kraftsow and the American Viniyoga Institute (AVI); Desikachar has expanded his approach

52

in conjunction with his son Kausthub under the new umbrella of The Krishnamacharya Healing and Yoga Foundation (KHYF), headquartered in Chennai (formerly Madras), India. As the teacher of well-known Yoga masters B.K.S. Iyengar, K. Pattabhi Jois, and Indra Devi, Professor T.S. Krishnamacharya can be said to have launched a veritable Hatha Yoga renaissance in modern times that is still sweeping the world.

✔ **Ashtanga Yoga** originated with Shri Krishnamacharya and was taught by K. Pattabhi Jois, who was born in 1915 but who had a suitably modern outlook to draw eager Western students to his Mysore, India, Ashtanga Yoga Institute until his death in 2009. He was a principal disciple of T.S. Krishnamacharya, who apparently instructed him to teach the sequences known as Ashtanga Yoga or Power Yoga. This style is by far the most athletic of the three versions of Hatha Yoga, going back to T.S. Krishnamacharya, and it combines postures with breathing. Ashtanga Yoga differs from Patanjali's eightfold path (also called Ashtanga Yoga), though it's theoretically grounded in it. (We discuss the Ashtanga Yoga tradition in "Considering Your Options: The Eight Main Branches of Yoga" earlier in this chapter.)

Power Yoga is a generic term for any style that follows closely Ashtanga Yoga but doesn't have a set series of postures. It emphasizes flexibility and strength and was mainly responsible for introducing Yoga postures into gyms. Beryl Bender Birch, Bryan Kest, Baron Baptiste, and Sherri Baptiste Freeman are all closely associated with Power Yoga. In a similar manner, *Vinyasa Yoga* and *Flow Yoga*, developed by Ganga White and Tracey Rich, are also variatons of Ashtanga Yoga.

- **Anusara Yoga,** with strong roots in Iyengar Yoga, has attained great popularity within a short span of time. Created in 1997 by the American Yoga teacher John Friend, its appeal is in its heart-centered approach. Based on the three *A*s — attitude, alignment, and action — Anusara Yoga seeks to bring "grace" *(anusara)* into a posture and thus give Hatha Yoga a spiritual thrust.

- **Kripalu Yoga,** inspired by Swami Kripalvananda (1913–1981) and developed by his disciple Yogi Amrit Desai, is a three-stage Yoga tailored for the needs of Western students. The first stage emphasizes postural alignment and coordination of breath and movement; you hold the postures for a short time only. The second stage adds meditation and prolongs the postures. In the final stage, practicing the postures becomes a spontaneous meditation in motion. See Chapter 24 for more information about the Kripalu Yoga Center in Massachusetts.

- **Integral Yoga** was developed by Swami Satchidananda (1914–2002), a student of the famous Swami Sivananda of Rishikesh, India. Swami Satchidananda made his debut at the Woodstock festival in 1969, where he taught the baby boomers to chant *om,* and over the years has attracted thousands of students. As the name suggests, this style aims to integrate the various aspects of the body-mind through a combination of postures, breathing techniques, deep relaxation, and meditation. Chapter 24 gives you more information about the Satchidananda Ashram in Virginia.

✔ **Sivananda Yoga** is the creation of the late Swami Vishnudevananda (1927–1993), also a disciple of Swami Sivananda of Rishikesh, India, who established his Sivananda Yoga Vedanta Center in Montreal in 1959. He trained over 6,000 teachers, and you can find numerous Sivananda centers around the world. This style includes a series of 12 postures, the Sun Salutation sequence, breathing exercises, relaxation, and *mantra* chanting.

✔ **Ananda Yoga** is anchored in the teachings of Paramahansa Yogananda (1893–1952) and was developed by Swami Kriyananda (Donald Walters), one of his disciples. This gentle style prepares the student for meditation, and its distinguishing features are the silent affirmations associated with holding the postures. This Yoga style includes Yogananda's unique energization exercises, first developed in 1917, which involve consciously directing the body's energy (life force) to different organs and limbs. You can find more information about the Ananda Institute of Alternative Living in Nevada City, California, in Chapter 24.

✔ **Kundalini Yoga** isn't only an independent approach of Yoga but also the name of a style of Hatha Yoga, originated by the Sikh master Yogi Bhajan (1929–2004). Its purpose is to awaken the serpent power *(kundalini)* by means of postures, breath control, chanting, and meditation. Yogi Bhajan, who came to the United States in 1969, is the founder and spiritual head of the Healthy, Happy, Holy Organization (3HO), which has headquarters in Los Angeles and numerous branches

55

around the world. (We cover the Kundalini Yoga approach in the earlier section "Considering Your Options: The Eight Main Branches of Yoga.")

✔ **Hidden Language Yoga** was developed by the late Swami Sivananda Radha (1911–1995), a German-born female student of Swami Sivananda. This style seeks to promote not only physical well-being but also self-understanding by exploring the symbolism inherent in the postures. Hidden Language Yoga is taught by the teachers of Yasodhara Ashram in British Columbia (see Chapter 24).

✔ **Somatic Yoga** is the creation of Eleanor Criswell, EdD, a professor of psychology at Sonoma State University in California who has taught Yoga since the early 1960s. Somatic Yoga is an integrated approach to the harmonious development of body and mind, based both on traditional yogic principles and modern psychophysiological research. This gentle approach emphasizes visualization, very slow movement into and out of postures, conscious breathing, mindfulness, and frequent relaxation between postures.

✔ **Moksha Yoga,** which was originally based on the style of Bikram Yoga (in the following bullet) and is popular in Canada, uses traditional postures in a heated room and includes relaxation periods. It champions a green philosophy.

✔ **Bikram Yoga** is the style taught by Bikram Choudhury. Bikram Choudhury, who achieved fame as the teacher of Hollywood stars, teaches at the Yoga College of India in Bombay and other locations around the world, including San Francisco and Tokyo. This style, which has a set routine of

26 postures, is fairly vigorous and requires a certain fitness level for participation, especially because it calls for a high room temperature.

You also may hear or see a mention of other Yoga styles, including Tri Yoga (developed by Kali Ray), White Lotus Yoga (developed by Ganga White and Tracey Rich), Jivamukti (developed by Sharon Gannon and David Life), Ishta Yoga (an acronym for the Integrated Science of Hatha, Tantra, and Ayurveda, developed by Mani Finger), Forrest Yoga (a mixture of Hatha Yoga and Native American ideas created by Ana Forrest), and Prime of Life Yoga (developed by me [Larry]) for midlife and beyond.

Hot Yoga isn't really a style itself; it just means that the practice occurs in a high-temperature room (90 to 100 degrees Fahrenheit). It usually refers to either Ashtanga Yoga or Bikram Yoga.

Finding Your Niche: Five Basic Approaches to Yoga

Since Yoga came to the Western hemisphere from its Indian homeland in the late 19th century, it has undergone various adaptations. Today, Yoga is practiced in five major ways:

- ✔ As a method for physical fitness and health maintenance

- ✔ As a sport

- ✔ As body-oriented therapy

- ✔ As a comprehensive lifestyle

- ✔ As a spiritual discipline

The first three approaches are often grouped into the category of Postural Yoga, which is contrasted with Traditional Yoga (the final two bullets). As its name suggests, Postural Yoga focuses (sometimes exclusively) on Yoga postures. Traditional Yoga seeks to adhere to the traditional teachings as taught anciently in India. We take a look at the five basic approaches in the upcoming sections.

Yoga as fitness training

The first approach, Yoga as fitness training, is the most popular way that Westerners practice Yoga. It's also the most radical revamping of Traditional Yoga. More precisely, it's a modification of traditional Hatha Yoga. Yoga as fitness training is concerned primarily with the physical body's flexibility, resilience, and strength. Fitness is how most newcomers to Yoga encounter this great tradition. Fitness training is certainly a useful gateway into Yoga, but later on, some people discover that Hatha Yoga is a profound *spiritual* tradition. From the earliest times, Yoga masters have emphasized the need for a healthy body. But they've also always pointed beyond the body to the mind and other vital aspects of the being.

Yoga as a sport

Yoga as a sport is an especially prominent approach in some Latin American countries. Its practitioners, many of whom are excellent athletes, master hundreds of extremely difficult Yoga postures to perfection and demonstrate their skills and beautiful physiques in international competitions. But this new sport, which also can be regarded as an art form, has drawn much criticism from the ranks of more traditional Yoga practitioners who feel that competition has no place in Yoga. Yet this athletic orientation has done much to put Yoga on the map in some parts of the world, and we see nothing wrong with good-natured Yoga "competitions" as long as participants hold self-centered competitiveness in check.

The increasingly popular fad of Acro-Yoga, which specializes in acrobatic moves done in combination with a partner, also falls into the Yoga-as-a-sport category. Only the fittest and most flexible are able to practice this modern variation of Yoga without risk of injury. However, purists find fault with the lack of spiritual and ethical intention behind this style of Hatha Yoga.

Yoga as therapy

The third approach, Yoga as therapy, applies yogic techniques to restore health or full physical and mental function. In recent years, some Western Yoga teachers have begun to use yogic practices for therapeutic purpose. Although the idea behind Yoga therapy is very old, its name is fairly new. In fact, Yoga therapy is a whole new professional discipline, calling for far greater training and skill on the part of the teacher than is the case with ordinary Yoga. Commonly, Yoga is intended for those who don't suffer from disabilities or ailments requiring remedial action and special attention. Yoga therapy, on the other hand, addresses these special needs. For example, Yoga therapy may be able to help you find relief from many common ailments. Chapter 22 of this book shows you some basic yogic techniques for improving common lower and upper back problems.

Yoga as a lifestyle

Yoga as a lifestyle enters the proper domain of Traditional Yoga. Yoga once or twice a week for an hour or so is certainly better than no Yoga at all. And Yoga can be enormously beneficial even when practiced only as fitness training or as so-called Postural Yoga. But you unlock the real potency of Yoga when you adopt it as a lifestyle — *living* Yoga and practicing it every day whether through physical exercises or meditation. Above all, you apply the wisdom of Yoga to everyday life and live *lucidly,* with awareness. Yoga has much to say about what and how you should eat, how you should sleep, how you should work, how you should relate to others, and so on. It offers a total system of conscious and skillful living.

In modern times, a Yoga lifestyle includes caring for the ailing environment, an idea especially captured in Green Yoga. (Check out the sidebar "Healing the planet through Green Yoga" in this chapter for more information.) Don't think you have to be a yogic superstar to practice lifestyle Yoga. You can begin today. Just make a few simple adjustments in your daily schedule and keep your goals vividly in front of you. Whenever you're ready, make further positive changes one step at a time. See Chapter 20 for more on working Yoga into your whole day.

Yoga as a spiritual discipline

Lifestyle Yoga (see the preceding section) is concerned with healthy, wholesome, functional, and benevolent living. Yoga as a spiritual discipline, the fifth and final approach, is concerned with all that *plus* the traditional ideal of *enlightenment* — that is, discovering your spiritual nature. This approach is often equated with Traditional Yoga. (We discuss the journey to enlightenment in Chapter 21.)

The word *spiritual* has been abused a lot lately, so we need to explain how we use it here. *Spiritual* relates to *spirit* — your ultimate nature. In Yoga, it's called the *atman* (pro-

60

nounced *aht-mahn*) or *purusha (poo-roo-shah)*.

According to nondualistic (based in one reality) Yoga philosophy, the *spirit* is one and the same in all beings and things. It's formless, immortal, superconscious, and unimaginably blissful. It's transcendental because it exists beyond the limited body and mind. You discover the spirit fully in the moment of your enlightenment.

What most approaches to Yoga have in common

Most traditional or tradition-oriented approaches to Yoga share two fundamental practices, the cultivation of awareness and relaxation:

- ✔ *Awareness* is the peculiarly human ability to pay close attention to something, to be consciously present, and to be mindful. Yoga is attention training. To see what we mean, try this exercise: Pay attention to your right hand for the next 60 seconds. That is, feel your right hand and do nothing else. Chances are, your mind is drifting off after only a few seconds. Yoga asks you to rein in your attention whenever it strays.

- ✔ *Relaxation* is the conscious release of unnecessary and therefore unwholesome tension in the body.

Both awareness and relaxation go hand in hand in Yoga. Without bringing awareness and relaxation to Yoga, the exercises are merely exercises — not *yogic* exercises.

Conscious breathing is often added to awareness and relaxation as a third foundational practice. Normally, breathing happens automatically. In Yoga, you bring awareness to this act, which then makes it into a powerful tool for training your body and your mind. We say much more about these aspects of Yoga in Chapter 5.

Health, Healing, and Yoga

The source of your health and happiness lies within you. Outside agents like physicians, therapists, or remedies can help you through major crises, but you yourself are primarily responsible for your own health and happiness. The following sections show you how Yoga helps you mobilize the inner strength to live responsibly and wisely.

What is health? Most people answer this question by saying that health is the opposite of illness, but *health* is more than the absence of disease — it's a positive state of being.

Something for nothing?

You get out of Yoga what you put into it. One computer term particularly relevant to Yoga practice is *gigo,* which means "garbage in, garbage out." It captures a simple truth: The quality of a cause determines the quality of the effect — what you get out of any endeavor is only as good as what you put in. In other words,

✔ Don't expect health from junk food.

✔ Don't expect happiness from miserable attitudes.

✔ Don't expect good results from shoddy Yoga practice.

✔ Don't expect something from nothing.

Yoga is a powerful tool, but you must learn to use it properly. You can buy the latest super-duper computer, but if you only know how to use it as a typewriter, that's all it is.

Health is wholeness. To be healthy means not only to possess a well-functioning body and a sane mind but also to vibrate with life, to be vitally connected with your social and physical environment. To be healthy also means to be happy.

Because life is constant movement, you shouldn't expect health to be static. Today health is increasingly difficult to achieve because the environment has become highly toxic. Perfect health is a mirage. In the course of your life, you can expect inevitable fluctuations in your state of health; even cutting your finger with a knife temporarily upsets the balance. Your body reacts to the cut by mobilizing all the necessary biochemical forces to heal itself. Regular Yoga practice can create optimal conditions for self-healing. You achieve a baseline of health, with an improved immune system that enables you to stay healthy longer and heal faster.

Yoga is about healing rather than curing. Like a really good physician, Yoga takes deeper causes into account instead of slapping a bandage on surface symptoms. These causes are more often than not found in the mind — in the way you live and how you think. That's why Yoga masters recommend self-understanding. Most people tend to be passive in health matters. They wait until something goes wrong and then rely on a pill or a physician to fix the problem. Yoga encourages you to take the initiative in preventing illness and restoring or maintaining your health. Taking control of your health has nothing to do with self-doctoring (which can be dangerous); it's simply a matter of taking responsibility for your health. A good physician can tell you that a patient's active participation in the process greatly facilitates healing. For example, you may take various kinds of medication to deal with a gastric ulcer, but unless you learn to eat well, sleep adequately, avoid stress, and take life more easily, you're bound to have a recurrence before long. You must change your lifestyle to realize any deep-seated healing.

Yoga points the way to happiness, health, and life-embracing meaning by suggesting that the best possible meaning you can find for yourself springs from the well of joy deep within you. That joy or bliss is the very nature of the spirit, or transcendental Self (refer to "Yoga as a spiritual discipline" earlier in this chapter). Joy is like a 3-D lens that captures life's bright colors and motivates you to embrace life in all its countless forms.

Balancing Your Life with Yoga

The Hindu tradition explains Yoga as the discipline of balance, another way of expressing the ideal of unity through Yoga. Everything in you must harmonize to function optimally. A disharmonious mind is disturbing in itself, but sooner or later it also causes physical problems. An imbalanced body can easily warp your emotions and thought processes. If you have strained relationships with others, you cause distress not only for them but also for yourself. And when your relationship to your physical environment is disharmonious, well, you trigger serious repercussions for everyone.

A beautiful and simple Yoga exercise called "The Tree" (described in Chapter 9) improves your sense of balance and promotes your inner stillness. Even when conditions force a tree to grow askew, it always balances itself out by growing a branch in the direction opposite its lean, so in this posture, you stand still like a tree, perfectly balanced.

Healing the planet through Green Yoga

The environmental crisis, which is sharpening day by day, is prompting more and more yogis and yoginis to apply Yoga's ethical standards specifically to the health of the ailing planet. This Green Yoga approach is explained in my (Georg's) and Brenda Feuerstein's book *Green Yoga* (Traditional Yoga Studies).

Green Yoga is Yoga that incorporates environmental mindfulness and activism in its spiritual orientation. It centers on a deep reverence for all life and a lifestyle of voluntary simplicity; it believes the time has come to make Yoga count in more than personal terms.

If you want to get started on greening your Yoga, try carpooling or biking to your next class, or use an environment-friendly Yoga mat. Also, reduce! Reuse! Recycle!

Yoga helps you apply this principle to your life. Whenever life's demands and challenges force you to bend to one side, your inner strength and peace of mind serve as counterweights. Rising above all adversity, you can never be uprooted.

Chapter 2

Ready, Set, Yoga!

In This Chapter

▶ Being clear about why you want to practice
▶ Finding the right Yoga style, class, and teacher (or lack thereof) for yourself
▶ Preparing for a Yoga session

This chapter gives you everything you need to prepare for your Yoga practice, whether you opt to take part in a class or practice solo. We discuss setting goals, getting the proper gear, finding enough time to practice, and more.

Make sure that you're physically ready before you begin this new venture with Yoga or any fitness activity. Consult with your doctor, especially if you have an existing health challenge. Even if your medical history includes experience with hypertension, heart problems, arthritis, or chronic back pain, you can benefit from Yoga. In more severe cases, you may want to work closely with a competent Yoga therapist to create just the right routines and to monitor your progress.

Setting a Goal for Your Practice

Before you start too far into considering classes and purchasing gear, first things first. Take a deep breath, exhale slowly, and then ask yourself: What do I want from my Yoga experience? Consider the following questions:

- Do I simply want to try Hatha Yoga because it's a trendy thing to do?

- Am I hoping to find a way to decompress (clear the mind and alleviate stress)?

- Is physical fitness my main interest?

- Do I simply want to have a more flexible body?

- Does meditation intrigue me?

- Do the spiritual aspects of Yoga interest me?

- Do I have health concerns, such as lower back problems or hypertension that I expect Yoga to help handle?

Obviously, if your goals are entirely spiritual, you must choose a branch of Yoga that can best help you achieve those goals. You may resonate with Bhakti Yoga, Jnana Yoga, Raja Yoga, Karma Yoga, or Tantra Yoga, all of which we introduce in Chapter 1. (Unfortunately, you also need to pick up a different book because this book is meant to primarily serve candidates of Hatha Yoga, which is the most popular branch in the West.) If your main interest is in improving your health or overall physical well-being, or you want to become fit and flexible, you have to select which style of Hatha Yoga fits you best (refer to Chapter 1 for more).

After you're clear about your motivation and expectations, don't just think it — ink it. Write down your goals so that you can really focus on your specific needs. For example, your *goal* may be to be able to better cope with stress. In order to achieve that goal, you have to take your particular *needs* into account. If you're a super-busy mom and have only half an hour of slack time at night during the week and perhaps a full hour on Sundays, your *need* is obviously to keep your Yoga program very simple.

No excuses, please

Most people are aware of how fast time flies in the 24 hours they're given each day. Yet if you look more closely at how you spend your days, you may find that not everything you do is necessary, and that in idle moments, you may miss the opportunity to recharge yourself or tap into your inner well of joy. If you've picked up this book and are reading these lines, chances are you have enough time to practice Yoga regularly.

If you think you're not capable of practicing Hatha Yoga because it requires too much flexibility or is otherwise too demanding physically, turn your attention to this truth: You can be as stiff as a board and still benefit from Yoga! The yogic postures help you become more flexible, whatever your starting point. Don't gauge yourself by the photos you may see in some Yoga books. They usually show advanced practitioners at their best. This book focuses on the needs of beginners. After you take the first few steps, the next big leap may not seem quite so challenging.

Checking Out Various Yoga Class Options

So, you're sure that you want to take the Yoga plunge. What's your safest bet? To put it plainly, set your sights on a suitable Yoga class or teacher instead of sailing away as a strict do-it-yourselfer. Although you can explore some basic practices by reading about them (this book makes sure of that!), a full-fledged, safe Yoga routine really requires proper instruction from a qualified teacher. The following sections help you determine what kind of class to seek out.

Many Yoga schools offer introductory courses (four to six weeks), so you don't have to jump into the deep end. After a few classes and the benefit of an instructor's expert advice, you can certainly continue practicing and exploring Yoga on your own (see the section "Skipping Class" later in this chapter). In that case, you may still want to check in with a teacher every so often, just to make sure that you haven't acquired any bad habits in executing the various postures and other practices.

Finding a class that's right for you

If you live in a big city, you're bound to have several choices for group classes, but if you live in a small town you may have to be more resourceful. Here are some suggestions for finding the Yoga class that's right for you:

- Tell your friends that you want to join a Yoga class; some of them may start raving about their classes or teachers.

- Consult the resources we list in the appendix.

- Look at bulletin boards in health food stores and adult education centers.

69

✔ Check online resources (see the appendix).

✔ Look into possibilities at your local health club, but before joining a Yoga session, make sure that the teacher is really qualified: How much training has he or she had? Is proper certification hanging on his or her office wall?

✔ Ask your local librarian.

✔ Head toward the back of the local phone book to check out listings under Yoga Instruction.

Checking out classes and teachers

We think that visiting a few places and teachers is important before committing to a course or a series of classes. Some Yoga schools give out the telephone numbers of their teachers, and you may want to have a phone conversation before making a special trip to the school. When you visit a Yoga center or classroom, pay attention to your intuitive feelings about the place. Consider how the staff treats you and how you respond to the people attending class. Stroll around the facility and feel its overall energy. First impressions are often (although not always) accurate. Some teachers even let you quietly look in on a class; others find this practice too distracting for their students.

 Bring a written checklist to your class visit. Don't feel embarrassed about being thorough. If you don't want to be so obvious, memorize the points that you want to check out. Here are some ideas for your list:

✔ How do I feel about the building or classroom's atmosphere?

✔ What's my gut response to the teacher?

- Do I want a male or female teacher?
- What are the teacher's credentials?
- Does the teacher or school have a good reputation?
- How do I respond to other students?
- Do the programs suit my needs?
- How big are the classes, and can I still get proper, individual attention from the teacher?
- Would I be happy coming here regularly?
- Can I afford the classes?

When checking out a Yoga center, don't hesitate to quiz the instructor or other staff members about any concerns. In particular, find out what style of Hatha Yoga they offer. Some styles — notably Ashtanga or Power Yoga — demand athletic fitness. Others embody a more relaxed approach. In this book, we favor the latter. However, we can readily appreciate that some vigorous people may feel attracted to and benefit from yogic routines that are the equivalent of a workout and that call for strength, endurance, high flexibility, and a drench of perspiration.

If you're not familiar with the style of a particular school, don't hesitate to ask for an explanation (check out our explanation of styles in Chapter 1). Yoga practitioners are usually pretty friendly folk, eager to answer your questions and put your mind at ease. If they aren't, put a mark in the appropriate box in your mental checklist. Remember that even nice people, including Yoga practitioners, can have occasional off-days. But if you don't feel welcome and comfortable on your first visit, you probably won't receive better treatment later on.

What makes a good teacher?

A good Yoga teacher should be an example of what Yoga is all about: a balanced person who isn't only skillful in the postures but also courteous and thoughtful toward others and adaptive and attentive to everyone's individual needs in class. Check out the teacher's credentials to be sure that he or she has been properly trained or is certified in one of the established traditions. Consult Chapter 23 and the appendix for our recommendations on some of the well-established larger Yoga organizations.

We caution you to steer clear of teachers who have taken only a few workshops on Yoga or received their diplomas in a three-day course. They may be excellent aerobics instructors who know nothing about Yoga. Also avoid the drill sergeant type or anyone who makes you feel intimidated about your level of skill in performing the postures. By the way, under no circumstances allow your instructor to push or coerce you into a posture that doesn't feel right or that causes you pain.

Making sure courses fit your experience level

If you're a beginner, look for a beginner's course. You're likely to feel more comfortable in a group that's starting at the same skill level instead of being surrounded by advanced practitioners who can perform difficult postures easily and elegantly. Whatever the skill level of a class, don't feel self-conscious. None of the advanced students will stare at you to see whether the new kid in class is any good. You may get a few encouraging smiles, though.

 Beginner classes are sometimes advertised as *Easy Does It Yoga* or *Gentle Yoga.*

As a beginner, be leery of overly large classes (more than 20 students) or mixed-level classes that lump together Yoga freshmen with postgraduates. Your teacher can't give you the attention you deserve to ensure your safety. Keep in mind, though, that many of the more experienced teachers are quite popular, and their classes tend to be large; you may have to decide whether personal attention or a higher level of teacher experience is more important to you.

Public or private?

Decide whether you want to learn Hatha Yoga in a group or from a private instructor. In practice, most people start with a group class because of the cost and the boost in motivation that comes from practicing with other people. If you can afford private lessons, however, even a few sessions can be extremely beneficial. Importantly, if you have a serious health challenge, you need to work privately with a Yoga therapist (see the appendix for a list of organizations specializing in Yoga therapy).

Backyard studios and home classes

Throughout the world, many Yoga teachers hold sessions in their homes or in backyard studios. Don't let this practice turn you off — you may find a great opportunity. Some of the most dedicated Yoga teachers work this way because they want to avoid commercialism and the details of administering a full-scale center. Backyard studios often offer a great sense of community, and you can also expect lots of valuable, personal attention from the teacher because the groups tend to be smaller than those in larger centers.

Here's a sampling of the advantages of private lessons:

- ✔ You get personalized attention.
- ✔ You have the opportunity to interact more with the teacher during class.
- ✔ Your routines can vary more, with proper supervision.
- ✔ You can work more intensively with those exercises that are more challenging for you.
- ✔ If you're shy or easily distracted, you don't have to worry about the company of other people.

Here are a few advantages of group practice:

- ✔ You experience the support of the group.
- ✔ Your motivation is strengthened by seeing others succeed.
- ✔ You can make good, like-minded friends.
- ✔ Group sessions are easy on your pocketbook.

Checking the time: How long does a Yoga class last?

The length of a group Yoga class varies from 50 to 90 minutes. Health clubs, fitness spas, and corporate classes are normally 50 to 60 minutes long, but beginning classes at Yoga centers usually last from 75 to 90 minutes long. A private Yoga lesson customarily lasts one hour.

Paying the price: How much should a Yoga class cost?

In general, group Yoga classes are pretty affordable. The cheapest classes are usually available at adult education centers and community and senior centers. YMCA and YWCA classes also tend to be reasonably priced, or your health club may even include free Yoga classes as part of a fitness package. Most regular Yoga centers in metropolitan areas, however, charge on average $10 to $15 per class. A one-time drop-in fee (for those who haven't committed to taking more than one class) is usually a couple of dollars higher. Some schools offer the first class free, and others charge as much as $25.

You can do your own pricing research by phone and computer. More and more Yoga sites advertise on the Internet (see the appendix). They usually don't mention fees, but they do provide you with an e-mail address or a phone number. When you're considering a commitment to a Yoga center, check into the larger packages — they're often a good investment. Obviously, private lessons are quite a bit more expensive than group classes and range from $50 to $150.

Whenever you smell commercialism, you can be fairly sure your nose isn't deceiving you. If you're uncomfortable with the price you're quoted for Yoga classes, just search out a more reasonable offer. Here and there, you can even find free-of-charge classes, notably in Canada. Who said you can't get a free ride?

Going co-ed

Most Yoga classes welcome both genders, with an average ratio of seven women to three men enrolled in any session. Some of the more physically demanding styles of Hatha

Yoga, however, attract an equal number of athletic men and women.

Dressing for Success, and Other Yoga Practicing Considerations

After you choose a class you think can work for you, you may be nervous about actually taking the plunge and heading to your first session. The following sections aim to answer your questions about what to wear and take and how to stay safe (and in the good graces of your classmates) as you begin your group Yoga journey.

Deciding what to wear

Yoga practitioners wear a wide variety of exercise clothing. Practically speaking, what people wear depends on the difficulty level of the class and the temperature of the room. Of course, personal expression is also a consideration. A handful of eccentric groups practice in the nude, which really isn't a good idea because it's bound to distract some folks. Besides, you can easily catch a chill. Even when you practice on your own, you may want to cover your lower trunk to protect your kidneys and abdomen. At least that's the traditional Yoga way.

Women often wear leotards, sweats, shorts, and tops. Men usually wear shorts, sweats, T-shirts, and tank tops.

The key is to wear clean, comfortable, and decent clothes that allow you to move and breathe freely. Some people want to be fashionable by wearing the latest attention-drawing outfits, but we discourage this attitude. Simple does it!

If you're practicing outdoors or in a poorly heated room, you may want to layer your clothing so that you can peel off a layer when you're getting too warm from your Yoga practice. Also, extra clothing can come in handy when you get to the relaxation or meditation part of the class.

Packing your Yoga kit

Before attending a class, find out what kind of floor it practices on. If the floor is carpeted, a towel or a sticky mat works (we describe sticky mats and similar useful items in Chapter 19). A hardwood floor may require more padding, especially if your knees are sensitive. In that case, bring along a thick Yoga mat or a rug remnant that is a little longer than your height and a little wider than your shoulders. If you have a tendency to get cold, bring a blanket to cover yourself during final relaxation. A folded blanket is also helpful if you need a pad under your head when you're lying down. As your teacher becomes familiar with your unique needs, he or she may suggest some other personalized props for you to bring to class. As we discuss in Chapter 1, some Yoga styles — notably Iyengar Yoga — work more with props than others. Following are some general items you may want to bring to class with you:

- Your own Yoga mat or rug

- A towel

- A blanket

- Extra clothing to layer on if the room is too cool or to take off if you're too warm

- Bottled water (to balance your electrolytes after the session); we recommend that you use a steel flask with your own filtered water

✔ Enthusiasm, motivation, and good humor

If you're serious about your Yoga practice (and if you're concerned about hygiene), we recommend that you invest in your own personal mat and other equipment. Although many Yoga centers furnish this stuff, consider bringing your own. If you ever have to pick from the bottom of the bin after yet another sweaty class, you'll know what we mean.

Putting safety first

The most important factor for determining the safety of a Yoga class is your personal attitude. If you participate with the understanding that you aren't competing against the other students or the teacher and that you also must not inflict pain upon yourself, you can enjoy a safe Yoga practice. The popular maxim "No pain, no gain" doesn't really apply to Yoga. Perhaps "No gain with negative pain" is a better mindset.

By *negative pain,* we mean discomfort that causes you distress or increases the likelihood of injury. Of course, if you haven't exercised for a while, you can expect to encounter your body's resistance at the beginning. You may even feel a little sore the next day, which just reflects your body's adjustment to the new adventure. The key to avoiding injury is to proceed gently. It's better to err on the side of gentleness than to face torn ligaments. A good teacher always reminds you to ease into the postures and work creatively with your body's physical resistance. Nonharming is an important moral virtue in Yoga — and observation toward all beings includes yourself!

If you have any physical limitations (recent surgeries, knee, neck, or back problems, and so on), be sure to inform the center and the teacher beforehand. In a classroom setting, instructors have to split their attention among several students; your upfront communication can help prevent personal injury.

If a teacher insists that you do an exercise or a routine that feels very uncomfortable or that you feel may hurt you, take a break on your mat or, if that isn't possible, just walk out of the class. Try to stay cool and register your complaint with the school afterward. Fortunately, this situation rarely happens.

Paging Miss Manners

In all social settings, common courtesy calls for sensitivity to others; those same rules of responsible conduct apply to your participation in Yoga group sessions. So, sift through

Making time for Yoga

For centuries, the traditional time for Yoga practice has been sunrise and sunset, which are thought to be especially auspicious. These days, busy lifestyles can toss out lots of obstacles to your best intentions, so be pragmatic and arrange your Yoga practice at your convenience. Just keep in mind that statistically, you have a 30 percent greater chance of accomplishing a fitness goal if you practice in the morning. More important than holding tight to a preset time is just making sure that you work Yoga into your schedule *somewhere* — and stick with it.

Practicing at roughly the same time during the day can help you create a positive habit, which may make it easier to maintain your routine.

all the good manners you've accumulated from a lifetime of human interaction, and pack them as required equipment for your next trip to class. Before you go, check your bags for these etiquette essentials:

- ✔ Show up on time; don't wander into class "fashionably" late. It's rude and disturbing to others.

- ✔ If you show up early and students from the class before are still relaxing or meditating, respect their quiet time until your own session formally begins.

- ✔ Leave your shoes, chewing gum, cellphones, pagers, and crummy attitudes outside the classroom.

- ✔ Avoid smoking cigarettes or drinking alcohol before class.

- ✔ Bathe and take a restroom break before your Yoga session.

- ✔ Keep classroom conversation to a minimum — some people arrive early to meditate or to just sit quietly.

- ✔ Be sure to take your socks off if you practice on a slippery surface (just don't leave them near your neighbor's face). If you're self-conscious about your feet ("those ugly things"), remember that their 26 bones do a great job at propping up your body all day long. Besides, everyone else is far too busy to focus on your feet.

- ✔ Avoid excessive, clanky jewelry.

- ✔ Be sure that your, ahem, private parts are appropriately covered if you choose to wear loose-fitting shorts or, against our advice, super-tight outfits.

- ✔ Don't wear heavy perfume or cologne.

- Cut back on your garlic consumption on the day that you go to class.

- Sit near the door or window if you require a lot of air.

- Sit close to the instructor if you have hearing difficulties; many teachers speak softly to generate the right mood.

- If you have used any props in class, put them away neatly.

- Pay your teacher on time, without having to be reminded.

Skipping Class

Traditionally, Yoga is passed down from teacher to student. However, a few accomplished yogis and yoginis are self-taught. These independent spirits set a precedent for those who enjoy exploring new territory on their own. If you live in an isolated area and don't have easy access to a Yoga instructor or class, don't be disheartened. You still have several choices that can help you begin your yogic journey (and in the appendix we provide you with a fairly extensive list of resources). Here's an abbreviated version:

- Audiocassettes
- Books
- CDs
- DVDs
- Magazines
- Newsletters

- Newspapers
- Television
- Videos

Because Yoga is a motor skill, most people without access to a teacher rely on a DVD or video for instruction. If you opt for this particular approach, we recommend that you learn a routine and then begin listening only to the instructor's voice rather than focusing on the screen. Yoga emphasizes more inner work than outer activity; watching the screen interferes with this process. Listening to a disembodied voice works better. According to Yoga, the eye is an active and even aggressive sense, whereas the ear is a more passive receptor. That's why CDs and audiotapes can also work well, provided they're accompanied by informative illustrations.

We prefer a good Yoga book over magazine or newspaper articles, simply because the creation of a book usually requires more in-depth, detailed consideration of subject matter and presentation. Plus, they have fewer advertisements taking up valuable space than periodicals do. Look for our book recommendations in the appendix. But don't discount the value of a newsletter from a backyard Yoga studio, especially if it comes to you via the electronic ether. The publication can be a real find if it comes from a legitimate source.

The difficulty with self-tutoring at the beginning is that you may have trouble judging good form from bad form. You need time to understand how your body responds to the challenge of a posture and determine the proper correction for your body's own optimal form. Some people use a mirror to check the postures, but that only tells one side of the story and, more importantly, it externalizes the whole process too much.

Become comfortable with checking from the inside, through inwardly *feeling* your body. Until you're proficient at doing so, seek out a competent instructor if at all possible. He or she sees you objectively — from all sides — and can thus give you valuable feedback about your body's specific resistances and requirements.

Being a Committed Yogi or Yogini

The traditional practice time for Yoga is 24 hours a day, as we discuss in Chapter 20. But even full-fledged yogis and yoginis don't perform postures and other similar exercises for more than a few hours daily. (Of course, some of them don't practice any physical exercises at all but pursue meditation exclusively.) Some people can carve out a regular Yoga practice time in their daily schedules. Many others, however, find this commitment completely impractical. Yet you can still benefit by attending classes just twice a week; even attending a group session once a week may introduce a little balance into a hectic lifestyle. You also have many opportunities during the day to work in a few Yoga postures or breathing exercises — during car rides or coffee breaks, or while going shopping.

How much time you allocate to your postural practice depends entirely on your goals and lifestyle. Inevitably, the busier you are with work, chores around the house, and social life, the less time you have available for Yoga. Consider starting with twice a week for a minimum of 15 minutes and see whether you can build to 30 minutes as a realistic goal in the first three months. If you're able to dedicate more time to Yoga, try to practice daily. But set a realistic goal for yourself so that you don't stress-out about Yoga or give up on it before you're able to enjoy its benefits. Also, remember that even if you don't have much time during the week, you can apply what you learn from each session anytime and anywhere!

The amount of time that you dedicate to Yoga is a personal choice — no need to feel guilty about your decision. Guilt is counterproductive and has no place in Yoga practice.

Eating before Yoga practice

Whether you're taking a Yoga class or practicing on your own, the guidelines for eating before Yoga practice are similar to the advice given for most physical activities. With even the lightest meal, such as fruit or juice, allow at least one hour before class. For larger meals with vegetables and grains, allow two hours and for heavy meals with meat, three to four hours. Eating right after class is okay. You may even have worked up a good appetite.

Chapter 3

Prep Before Pep: Ensuring a Fruitful Yoga Practice

In This Chapter

▶ Approaching Yoga with a healthy attitude
▶ Leaving the competition behind
▶ Translating your own mind-body language
▶ Doing it your way without regret

In Yoga, *what* you do and *how* you do it are equally important, and both mind and body contribute to your actions. Yoga respects the fact that you aren't merely a physical body but a psychophysical *body-mind*. Full mental participation in even the simplest of physical exercise enables you to tap into your deeper potential as a human being.

This chapter is about cultivating the right attitude toward your Yoga practice, which is the best preparation for success in Yoga. We encourage you to find your own pace without pushing yourself and risking injury, and to leave your competitive spirit to other endeavors. We also emphasize function over form, proposing that a modified version of the "ideal form" of a posture that suits your needs

85

is the right form for you. Yoga is a creative endeavor that asks you to call upon the powers of your own mind as you explore and enjoy the possibilities.

Cultivating the Right Attitude

Attitudes are enduring tendencies in your mind that show themselves in your behavior as well as your speech. Yoga encourages you to examine all your basic attitudes toward life to discover which ones are dysfunctional so that you can replace them with more appropriate ones.

One attitude worth cultivating is balance in everything, which is a top yogic virtue. A balanced attitude in this context means that you're willing to build up your Yoga practice step by step instead of expecting instant perfection. It also means not basing your practice on incorrect assumptions, including the notion that Yoga is about tying yourself in knots. On the contrary, Yoga loosens all your

What's in a number?

The traditional Sanskrit texts of Hatha Yoga state that 8.4 million postures exist, which correspond to as many species of living creatures. Of these, it's said, only 84 are useful to humans, and 32 are especially important.

The number 84 has symbolic value and is the product of 12×7. The number 12 represents the fullness of a chronological cycle (as in the 12 months of the year, or the 12 signs of the zodiac). The number 7 stands for structural fullness (as in the 7 energy centers or *cakras* of the human body — see Chapter 20).

bodily, emotional, and intellectual knots. The following sections give you some guidelines for getting in the right Yoga mindset.

Leave pretzels for snack time

Many people are turned off when they see magazine covers showing photographs of experts in advanced postures with their limbs tied in knots. What these publications may fail to disclose is that most of these yogis and yoginis have practiced Yoga several hours a day for many years to achieve their level of skill. Trust us! You don't have to be a pretzel to experience the undeniable benefits of Yoga. The benefit you derive from Yoga is from practicing at a level appropriate for you and not from striking an advanced and "ideal" form.

More than 2,000 postures are possible in Yoga sports, one of five approaches we mention in Chapter 1; however, many of these poses call for such great strength and flexibility that only a top gymnast can perform them competently. Though these postures may look beautiful when mastered, they offer no greater health benefits than the 20 or so fundamental postures that make up most practitioners' daily routines. So, unless you aim to participate in Yoga competitions, don't worry about all those glamorous-looking postures. Most are new inventions, whereas Yoga masters have been content for centuries with just a handful of practices that have stood the test of time.

Practice at your own pace

Some people are natural pretzels. If you (like most) aren't inherently noodle-like, regular practice can increase your flexibility and muscular strength. We advocate a graduated approach. In Chapters 6 through 13, you can find all the preparatory and intermediary steps that lead up to the final forms for the various postures. The late Yoga master T.S. Krishnamacharya of Chennai (Madras), India, the source of most of the best-known orientations of modern Hatha Yoga, emphasized tailoring Yoga instruction to the needs of each individual and advised Yoga teachers to take into account a student's age, physical ability, emotional state, and occupation. We agree and offer this sound advice: Proceed gently, but steadfastly.

Note: If you like to learn Yoga from books, choose carefully. Do the exercise descriptions include all the stages of developing comfort with a particular posture? To ask a middle-aged newcomer to Yoga to imitate the final form of many of the postures without providing suitable transitions and adaptations is a prescription for disaster. For instance, in almost every book on Hatha Yoga — except ours — you see the headstand featured quite prominently. This posture has become something of a symbol for Yoga in the West. Headstands are powerful postures, to be sure, but they also count among the more advanced practices. Because this beginner's book emphasizes exercises that are both feasible and safe, we've chosen not to include the headstand. We say more about this decision in Chapter 10, which introduces safe inversion practices. Instead, we give you several adaptations that are easier to perform and have no risk attached to them.

Send the scorekeeper home

American children often grow up in a highly competitive environment. From childhood on, they're pressured to do more, push harder, and win. Young athletes grow up with the spirit of competitiveness. Although competition has its place in society, this type of competitive behavior has no place in the practice of Yoga.

Yoga is about peace, tranquility, and harmony — the exact opposite of the competitive mindset. Yoga doesn't require you to fight against anyone, least of all yourself, or to achieve some goal by force. On the contrary, you're invited to be kind to yourself and others and, above all, to collaborate with your body rather than coerce it or do battle with your mind.

Heed our cautionary tale: Many years ago, a middle-aged man came to one of our classes. He was a friendly enough fellow but extremely competitive and hard on himself. He announced right away that he was intent on mastering the lotus posture within a few weeks and pushed himself to do so during our classes. We urged him repeatedly to proceed more slowly. After only a few visits, he failed to show up and never returned. Later, we learned from a mutual friend that in his competitive zeal, he had asked his wife to sit on his legs to force them into the lotus posture. Her weight had seriously injured both his knees!

No pain, no gain — NOT!

The idea of *no pain, no gain* — a completely mistaken notion — often reinforces competitiveness. Although pain and discomfort are part of life, you don't have to invite them. Yoga doesn't ask you to be a masochist. On the contrary, the goal of Yoga is to overcome all suffering. Therefore, never flog your body; always only coax it gently. Our motto is *no gain from pain.*

Picture yourself in the posture

We encourage you to use visualization in the execution of postures. For example, before you do the cobra, shoulder stand, or triangle, take ten seconds or so to visualize yourself moving into the final posture. Make your visualization as vivid as possible. Enlist the powers of your mind!

Enjoying a Peaceful Yoga Practice

As you travel through yogic postures, you begin to build awareness of the communications taking place between your body and mind. Do you feel peacefully removed from the raging storm of life around you, comfortable and confident with your strength, motion, and steadiness? Or are you painfully noting the slow passage of time, sensing a physical awkwardness or strain in your movements? Listen to your own rhythms and acknowledge their importance to help make your Yoga experience an expression of peace, calm, and security. And that positive message is what Yoga practice is all about.

Busting the perfect posture myth

Some modern schools of Hatha Yoga claim that they teach "perfect" postures that you can slip into as easily as a tailor-made suit. But how can the same posture be perfect for both a 15-year-old athlete and a 60-year-old retiree? Besides, these schools disagree among themselves about what constitutes a perfect posture. So, to spell it out, the perfect posture is a perfect myth.

As the great Yoga master Patanjali explained nearly 2,000 years ago, posture has only two requirements: A posture should be steady and easeful:

- **Steady posture:** A *steady* posture is a posture that you hold stable for a certain period of time. The key isn't freezing all movement, though. Your posture becomes steady when your mind is steady. As long as your thoughts run wild, including your negative emotions, your body also remains unsteady. As you become more skilled in self-observation, you begin to notice the ever-revolving carousel of your mind and become sensitive to the tension in your body. That tension is what Yoga means by *unsteadiness.*

- **Easeful posture:** A posture is *easeful* when it's enjoyable and enlivening rather than boring and burdensome. An easeful posture increases the principle of clarity — *sattva* — in you. But easefulness isn't slouching. *Sattva* and joy are intimately connected. The more *sattva* is present in your body-mind, the more relaxed and happy you will be.

Although Patanjali was thinking primarily, perhaps even exclusively, in terms of meditation postures, his formula applies to all postures equally.

Listening to your body

No one knows your body like you do. The more you practice Yoga, the better you can become at determining your limitations, as well as your strengths, with each posture. Each posture presents its own unique challenge. You want to feel encouraged to explore and expand your physical and emotional boundaries without risking strain or injury to yourself.

Some teachers speak of practicing at the *edge,* the point at which the intensity of a posture challenges you but doesn't cause you pain or unusual discomfort. The idea is to very slowly and carefully push that edge farther back and open up new territory. Cultivate self-observation and pay attention to the feedback from your body to be able to practice at the edge.

Each Yoga session is an exercise in self-observation without being judgmental. Listen to what your body is telling you. Train yourself to become aware of the signals that continually travel from your muscles, tendons, ligaments, bones, and skin to your brain. Be in dialogue with your body instead of indulging in a mental monologue that excludes bodily awareness. Pay particular attention to signals coming from your neck, lower back, jaw muscles, abdomen, and any known problem areas of your body.

To gauge the intensity of a difficult Yoga posture, use a scale from one to ten, with ten being your threshold for tolerable pain. Imagine a flashing red light and an alarm bell going off after you pass level eight. Notice the signals and heed them, particularly your breath. If your breathing becomes labored, it usually indicates that, figuratively speaking, you're going over the edge. You're the world's foremost expert on what your body is trying to tell you.

Beginners commonly experience trembling when holding certain Yoga postures. Normally, the involuntary motion is noticeable in the legs or arms and is nothing to worry about, as long as you aren't straining. The tremors are simply a sign that your muscles are working in response to a new demand. Instead of focusing on the feeling that you've become a wobbly bowl of jelly, lengthen your breath a little if you can and allow your attention to go deeper within. If the trembling starts to go off the Richter scale, either ease up a little or end the posture altogether.

Moving slowly but surely

All postural movements are intended for slow performance. Unfortunately, most people are usually on automatic with movements that tend to be unconscious, too fast, and not particularly graceful. Most people are generally unaware of their bodies, but yogic postures lead you to adopt a different attitude. Among the advantages of slow motion are

- ✔ Enhanced awareness, which enables you to listen to what your body is telling you and to practice at the edge.

- ✔ Safer practice. Slowing down lowers the risk of straining or spraining muscles, tearing ligaments, or overtaxing your heart.

- ✔ Quicker relaxation.

- ✔ Improved breathing and breathing stamina.

- ✔ Shared workload among more muscle groups.

For the best results, practice your postures at a slow, steady pace while calmly focusing on your breath and the postural movement (flip to Chapter 5 for more info on breathing and movement). Resist the temptation to speed up; rather, savor each posture. Relax and be present here and now. If your breathing becomes labored or you begin to feel fatigued, rest until you're ready to go on.

If you find yourself rushing through your program, pause and ask yourself, "Why the hurry?" If you're truly short on time, shorten your program and focus on fewer postures. But if you just can't shake the feeling of being pressured by time, consider postponing your Yoga session altogether and practice conscious breathing (which we discuss in Chapter 5) while you go about your other business.

If you're rushing through your program because you're feeling bored or generally distracted, pause and remind yourself why you're practicing Yoga in the first place. Renew your motivation by telling yourself that you have plenty of time to complete your session. Boredom is a sign that you're detached from your own bodily experience and aren't living in the present moment. Participate fully in the process. If you need more than a mental reminder, use one of the relaxation techniques that we describe in Chapter 4 to slow yourself down. As we explain in Chapter 5, full yogic breathing in one of the resting postures also has a wonderful calming effect.

Practicing function over form with Forgiving Limbs

In Yoga, as in life, function is more important than form. It's the function and not the form of the posture that gives you its benefits. Beginners, in particular need to adapt postures to enjoy their function and benefits right from the start.

We call one very useful adaptive device *Forgiving Limbs*. With Forgiving Limbs, you give yourself permission to slightly bend your legs and arms instead of keeping them fully extended. Bent arms and legs enable you to move your spine more easily, which is the focus of many postures and the key to a healthy spine.

For example, the primary mechanical function of a standing forward bend is to stretch your lower back. If you have a good back, take a moment to see what we mean in this adapted posture that's safe for beginners:

1. **Stand up straight and *without forcing anything*, bend forward and try to place your head on your knees with the palms of your hands on the floor (see Figure 3-1a) or hold the backs**

of your ankles.

Very few men or women can actually do this, especially beginners.

2. **Now stand up again, separate your feet to hip width, and bend forward, allowing your legs to bend until you can place your hands on the floor and almost touch your head to your knees (see Figure 3-1b).**

WARNING! When bending forward, be sure not to bounce up and down as most people are inclined to do. You're not a bungee cord!

As you become more flexible — and you will! — gradually straighten your legs until you can come closer to the ideal posture. A common lower back injury occurs when weekend warriors inspired by young, nubile instructors try to do the seated version of the straight-legged forward bend and push too far.

Figure 3-1:
Standing forward bend without and with Forgiving Limbs.

Chapter 4

Relaxed Like a Noodle: The Fine Art of Letting Go of Stress

In This Chapter

▶ Understanding and dealing with stress
▶ Relaxing the body through mental and physical exercises

Life in general — not merely modern life — is inherently stressful. Even an inanimate object such as a rock can experience an element of stress. Not all stress is bad for you, however. The question is whether that stress is helping you or killing you.

Psychologists distinguish between *distress* and *eustress* (good stress). Yoga can help you minimize distress and maximize good, life-enhancing stress. For example, a creative challenge that stimulates your imagination and fires your enthusiasm but doesn't cause you anxiety or lost sleep is a positive event. Even a joyous celebration is, strictly speaking, stressful, but the celebration isn't the kind of stress that kills you — at least not in modest doses. On the other hand, doing nothing and feeling bored to tears is a form of negative stress.

In this chapter, we talk about how you can control negative stress not only through various yogic-relaxation techniques but also by cultivating appropriate attitudes and habits.

The Nature of Stress

Stress is a fact of life. Some estimates indicate that 80 percent of all illnesses result from stress. Endocrinologist Hans Selye, who pioneered stress research, distinguished three phases of the stress syndrome: alarm, resistance, and exhaustion. *Alarm* can be a harmless activity like stepping from a warm house into the cold air or receiving an upsetting phone call. Both situations require the body to make an adjustment, which is a kind of *resistance*. When the demand on the body goes on for too long, the stage of *exhaustion* sets in, which can lead to a complete breakdown of the body and the mind — be it heart disease, hypertension, failure of the immune system, or mental illness.

Bad stress creates an imbalance in the body and the mind, causing you to tense your muscles and breathe in a rapid and shallow manner. Under stress, your adrenal glands work overtime and your blood becomes depleted of oxygen, which starves your cells. Constant stress triggers the fight-or-flight response, putting you in a chronic state of alertness that's extremely demanding on your body's energies.

Because of the relentless demands of modern life — work, noise, pollution, and so on — most people experience chronic stress. How can you deal with it efficiently? Yoga suggests a three-pronged solution:

- ✔ Correct stress-producing *attitudes*.

- ✔ Change *habits* that invite stress into your life.

✔ Release existing *tension* in the body on an ongoing basis.

 Stress can occur without any unpleasant stimulus. Even a birthday celebration can cause you stress, usually because of some hidden anxiety (like another year to mark off). Stress is cumulative and can creep up on you so gradually that it's imperceptible — until its acute and adverse symptoms manifest.

Correcting wrong attitudes

Yoga's integrated approach works with both the body and the mind, offering potent antidotes to just the sort of attitudes that make you prone to stress, especially egotism, extreme competitiveness, perfectionism, and the sense of having to accomplish everything right now and by yourself. In all matters, Yoga seeks to replace negative thoughts and attitudes with positive mental dispositions; it asks you to be kind to yourself. Yogic practice helps you understand that everything has its proper place and time.

If you, like so many stress sufferers, have a hard time asking for help, Yoga can give you a real appreciation that everyone is interdependent. If you're by nature distrustful of others, Yoga puts you in touch with that part of your psyche that naturally trusts life itself. It shows you that you don't need to feel as if you're under attack, because your real life — your spiritual identity — can never be harmed or destroyed.

Changing poor habits

Everything in the universe follows an ebb-and-flow pattern that you can count on. Seasons change, and newborn

Wherever ego, I go

The ultimate source of stress is the ego, or what the Yoga masters call the "I-maker" *(ahamkara),* from *aham* ("I") and *kara* ("maker"). From the perspective of Yoga, the ego is a mistaken notion in which people identify with their particular bodies rather than the universe as a whole. Consequently, they experience fear of death and attachment to the body and the mind. This attachment, which is the survival instinct, in turn gives rise to all those many emotions and intentions that make up the game of life. Keeping this artificial center — the ego — going is inherently stressful. The Yoga masters all agree that by relaxing the grip of the ego, you can experience greater peace and happiness. Happy letting go!

babies eventually become elderly adults. Yogic wisdom recommends that you adopt the same natural patterns into your personal life. You may spend much of your time being serious, but you need to play, too. In fact, you need to make time to *just be* with no expectations and no guilt. Taking time to just be is good for your physical and mental health. Work and rest, tension and relaxation belong together as balanced pairs.

Often, people desperately maintain a hectic schedule because they can't envision an alternative that includes time out. They fear what may happen if they slow down. But money and standard of living aren't everything, and the *quality* of your life is far more important. Besides, if stress undercuts your health, you have to go into low gear anyway, and your climb back to health may prove very costly. Yoga gives you a baseline of tranquility to deal with your fears effectively, providing that you engage it at the mental level and not just the physical level.

Your inner wisdom tells you that your body and mind are subject to change and that nothing in your environment permanently stays the same. Therefore, there's no point in anxiously clinging to anything. Yoga recommends that you constantly remember your spiritual nature, which is beyond the realm of change and ever blissful. However, it also asks you to care for others and the world you live in, but all the while appreciating that you can't step into the same river twice.

For example, if you're a mother, you love and take tender care of your children. But if you're also a yogini, you don't succumb to the stress-producing illusion that you *own* your children. Instead, you always remain aware of the fact that your sons and daughters have their own lives to live, which may turn out to be quite different from yours, and that all you can do is guide them as best you can.

Of course, you can do many practical things, which are described in books on stress management, to reduce stressful situations. These suggestions include not waiting until the last minute to start or finish projects, improving your communication with others, avoiding confrontations, and accepting that we live in an imperfect world.

 Your daily Hatha Yoga routine, especially the relaxation exercises, can help you extend the feeling of peacefulness or calmness beyond the session to the rest of the day. Pick some activities or situations that you repeat several times a day as reminders to consciously relax, such as when you go to the bathroom, wait at a traffic light, sit down, open or close a door, look at your watch, or hang up the telephone. Whenever you encounter these activities, exhale deeply and consciously relax, remembering the peaceful feeling evoked in your daily session.

Detach yourself

Yoga shows you how to cultivate the *relaxation response* throughout the day by letting go of your hold on things. This phrase was coined by Herbert Benson, MD, who was among the first to point out the hidden epidemic of hypertension (high blood pressure) as a result of stress. In his #1 national bestseller *The Relaxation Response* (Harper Paperbacks), he calls the relaxation response "a universal human capacity" and "a remarkable innate, neglected asset."

Yoga teaches you how to tap into that underused capacity of your own body-mind. The yogic equivalent of the relaxation response is *vairagya,* which means literally "dispassion" or "nonattachment." We call it "letting go." Feeling passionate about what you do (rather than having a lukewarm attitude) is good, but at the same time, you merely invite suffering when you become too attached to people, situations, and the outcome of your actions. For most people, this lesson is difficult to learn; it's pretty much a lifelong lesson. You can start any time, but the best time to begin is now.

Yoga recommends an attitude of inner detachment in all matters. This detachment doesn't spring from boredom, failure, fear, or any neurotic attitude but from inner wisdom. Unfortunately, you can't turn on some tap to pour forth wisdom whenever you want it. You must acquire wisdom, either bit by bit as life presents opportunities or deliberately through an intelligent study of the yogic tradition. The latter approach can involve listening directly to the teachings of bona fide masters or studying the same teachings in book form. Yoga's traditional teachings are contained in many books — all translated from the Sanskrit language for the benefit of contemporary students.

Releasing bodily tension

Yoga pursues tension release through all its many different techniques, including breathing exercises and postures, but especially relaxation techniques. The former are a form of *active* or *dynamic relaxation,* the latter are a form of *passive* or *receptive relaxation.*

Relaxation Techniques That Work

The Sanskrit word for relaxation is *shaithilya,* which is pronounced *shy-theel-yah* and means "loosening." It refers to the loosening of bodily and mental tension — all the knots that you tie when you don't go with the flow of life. These knots are like kinks in a hose that prevent the water from flowing freely. Keeping muscles in a constant alert state expends a great amount of your energy, which then is unavailable when you call upon your muscles to really function. Conscious relaxation trains your muscles to release their grip when you don't use them. This relaxation keeps the muscles responsive to the signals from your brain telling them to contract so that you can perform all the countless tasks of a busy day.

Tips for a successful relaxation practice

Relaxation isn't quite the same as doing nothing. Often, when you believe you're doing nothing, you're actually busy contracting unused muscles quite unconsciously. Relaxation is a conscious endeavor that lies somewhere between effort and noneffort. To truly relax, you have to understand and practice the skill.

Relaxation doesn't require any gadgets, but you may want to try the following:

✔ Practice in a quiet environment where you're unlikely to be disturbed by others or the telephone.

✔ Try placing a small pillow under your head and a large one under your knees for support and comfort in the *supine,* or lying, positions. Alternatively, fold up a blanket.

✔ Ensure that your body stays warm. If necessary, heat the room first or cover yourself with a blanket. Particularly avoid lying on a cold floor, which isn't good for your kidneys.

✔ Don't practice relaxation techniques on a full stomach.

Deep relaxation: The corpse posture

The simplest and yet the most difficult of all Yoga postures is the corpse posture *(shavasana,* from *shava* and *asana,* pronounced *shah-vah sah-nah),* also widely known as the dead posture *(mritasana,* from *mrita* and *asana).* This posture is the simplest because you don't have to use any part of your body at all, and it's the most difficult precisely because you're asked to do nothing whatsoever with your limbs. The corpse posture is an exercise in mind over matter. The only props you need are your body and mind.

If you're high-strung, *asana* practice helps make the corpse posture more easily accessible.

Here's how you do the corpse posture:

1. **Lie flat on your back, with your arms stretched out and relaxed by your sides, palms up (or whatever feels most comfortable).**

Place a small pillow or folded blanket under your head if you need one and another large one under your knees for added comfort.

2. **Close your eyes.**

   Check out Figure 4-1 for a look at the corpse posture.

3. **Form a clear intention to relax.**

   Some people find picturing themselves lying in white sand on a sunny beach helpful.

4. **Take a couple of deep breaths, lengthening exhalation.**

5. **Contract the muscles in your feet for a couple of seconds and then consciously relax them.**

   Do the same with the muscles in your calves, upper legs, buttocks, abdomen, chest, back, hands, forearms, upper arms, shoulders, neck, and face.

6. **Periodically scan all your muscles from your feet to your face to check that they're relaxed.**

   You can often detect subtle tension around the eyes and the scalp muscles. Also relax your mouth and tongue.

7. **Focus on the growing bodily sensation of no tension and let your breath be free.**

8. **At the end of the session, before opening your eyes, form the intention to keep the relaxed feeling for as long as possible.**

9. **Open your eyes, stretch lazily, and get up slowly.**

Practice 10 to 30 minutes; the longer the duration, the better. But watch out! Relaxing for too long can make you drowsy.

Ending relaxation peacefully

Allowing relaxation to end on its own is best — your body knows when it has benefited sufficiently and naturally brings you out of relaxation. However, if you have only a limited time for the exercise, set your mental clock to 15, 20, or however many minutes after closing your eyes as part of your intention.

If you need to have a sound to remind you to return to ordinary waking consciousness, make sure that your wristwatch or clock isn't so loud that it startles you and provokes a heavy surge of adrenaline.

Staying awake during relaxation

If it looks like you're going to fall asleep while doing the corpse posture, try bringing your feet closer together. Also, periodically pay attention to your breathing, making sure it's even and unforced. Catnaps are generally excellent; if you're experiencing insomnia, however, we suggest you save your sleep until you go to bed at night. (For good anti-insomnia exercises, check out "Relaxation before sleep" and "Insomnia buster" later in this section.) In any case, the benefits of conscious relaxation are more profound than any catnap. The beautiful thing about relaxation is that you're conscious throughout the experience and can control it to some extent. Through relaxation, you become more in touch with your own body, which benefits you throughout the day: You can detect stress and tension in your body more readily and then take remedial action. Also, you avoid the risk of feeling drowsy afterward because you inadvertently entered into a deeper sleep. Remember that sleep isn't necessarily relaxing. That's why people sometimes wake up feeling like they've done heavy work in their sleep.

Afternoon delight

When your energies flag in the afternoon, try the following exercise, which is a great stress buster. You can practice it at home or in a quiet place at the office. Just make sure that you can't be interrupted. For this exercise, you need a sturdy chair, one or two blankets, and a towel or an eye bag (see Chapter 19 for more on this additional yoga resource). Allow five to ten minutes.

1. **Lie on your back and put your feet up on the chair, which should face you (see Figure 4-2).**

   Make sure that your legs and back are comfortable. Your legs should be 15 to 18 inches apart. You can also put your legs and feet up on the edge of a bed. If none of the feet-up positions feels good, just lie on your back with your legs bent and feet placed on the floor. If the back of your head isn't flat on the floor, and your neck and throat feel tense, or if your chin is pushed up toward the ceiling, raise your head slightly on a folded blanket or firm flat cushion to feel comfortable.

106

Figure 4-2:
Lie on your back and put your feet on a chair.

2. **Cover your body from the neck down with one of the blankets.**

   Don't let your body cool down too quickly, which can not only feel uncomfortable and interfere with your relaxation but also cramp your muscles and harm your kidneys.

3. **Place the eye bag or towel folded lengthwise over your eyes.**

4. **Rest for a few moments and get used to the position.**

5. **Visualize a large balloon in your stomach. As you inhale through your nose, expand the imaginary balloon in all directions. As you exhale through your nose, release the air from the balloon.**

   Repeat this step several times until it becomes easy for you.

6. **Inhale freely and begin to make your exhalation longer and longer.**

   Inhale freely, exhale forever.

107

7. **Repeat Step 6 at least 30 times.**

8. **When you finish the exercise, allow your breath to return to normal and rest for a minute or so, enjoying the relaxed feeling.**

   Don't rush getting up.

Magic triangles

The following relaxation technique utilizes your power of imagination. If you can picture things easily in your mind, you may find the exercise enjoyable and refreshing. For this exercise, you need a chair and a blanket (if necessary). Allow five minutes.

1. **Sit up tall in a chair, with your feet on the floor and comfortably apart and your hands resting on top of your knees as shown in Figure 4-3.**

   If your feet aren't comfortably touching the floor, fold up the blanket and place it under your feet for support.

Figure 4-3:
Sit with your feet on the floor and your hands on your knees.

2. **Breathe through your nose but allow your**

108

breath to move freely.

3. **Close your eyes and focus your attention on the middle of your forehead, just above the level of your eyebrows.**

   Make sure that you don't crinkle your forehead or squint your eyes.

4. **Visualize as vividly as possible a triangle connecting the forehead point and the palms of both hands.**

   Register (but don't think about) any sensations or colors that appear on your mental screen while you hold the triangle in your mind. Do this visualization for 8 to 10 breaths and then dissolve the triangle.

5. **Visualize a triangle formed by your navel and the big toes of your feet.**

   Retain this image for 10 to 12 breaths. If any part of the mental triangle is difficult to connect, keep focusing on that part until the triangle fully forms.

6. **Keeping your eyes closed, visualize again the first triangle formed between your forehead and your two palms and then simultaneously visualize the second triangle (navel to toes).**

   This final step is more challenging. Picture both triangles together for 12 to 15 breaths and then dissolve them.

Relaxation before sleep

If you want to enjoy deep sleep or are experiencing insomnia (but don't want to count sheep), the following exercise can help you. Many people don't make it to the end of this relaxation technique without falling asleep. For this exercise, you need the following props: a bed or other comfortable place to sleep, two pillows, and one or two blankets. Allow five to ten minutes.

1. **Prepare yourself for sleep and get into bed, lying on your back under the blankets.**

   Your legs can be straight or bent at the knees with your feet flat on the mattress.

2. **Place one pillow or folded blanket under your head and have the other onc close by.**

3. **With your eyes closed, begin to breathe through the nose, making your exhalation twice as long as your inhalation.**

   Keep your breathing smooth and effortless. Also, don't try to direct your breath to any part of your body. Let the breathing pattern be effortless, something you can keep up.

4. **Remain on your back for eight breaths and then roll over onto your right side and place the second pillow between your knees.**

   Now use the same breathing ratio from Step 3 for 16 breaths.

5. **Finally, roll over on to your left side, with the second pillow still between your knees, and use the breathing ratio for 32 breaths.**

Insomnia buster

This exercise is for those who suffer from insomnia but have an active imagination. Instead of watching your mind weave tale after tale when you can't sleep at night, why not

Insomnia

Over 100 million North Americans suffer from chronic sleeplessness for medical, psychological, social, or environmental reasons. A medical cause may be a diagnosed or undiagnosed chronic disease, a temporary illness (such as the flu), pain, or reaction to a remedy. A psychological cause may be general anxiety, depression, anger, or alertness (such as expecting to be awakened by your baby). A social cause may be the habit of going to bed too late or having a late meal. An environmental cause may be a noisy neighborhood or a toxic home.

Obviously, you want to rule out interference from a chronic disease or reaction to a medication, so if need be, consult a physician or a pharmacist. You know whether you're anxious, depressed, or overly alert and whether your social habits are or aren't conducive to your sleep and well-being. But here are some sleep habits that represent their own obstacle to a good night's rest:

🖊 **Being fearful about insomnia by entertaining such misconceived notions that if you don't sleep eight hours every day you will die, go literally crazy, or become totally inefficient.** Generally, these extremes don't happen. These mental expectations program your body to fulfill your own prophecies. More often than not, insomniacs sleep many more hours than they think. Especially, older folks who swear that they haven't slept a wink in days can be found happily snoozing after lunch or another time during the day.

🖊 **Anxiously watching the clock.** The best thing is to place your clock where you can't see or reach it.

To combat insomnia, cultivate the following:

- ✔ **Make peace with yourself and everyone else when getting ready for sleep.** That's a good habit anyway.

- ✔ **Don't force yourself to sleep.** That's where knowing your personal *diurnal* (daytime) rhythm comes in handy. Some people are naturally sleepy by 9 p.m., but others have a few more hours of activity in them because they rise a bit later. If you go to bed two hours too early, you shouldn't be surprised if you just lie awake counting sheep. Acquaint yourself with your body's unique rhythm or, rather, rhythms.

- ✔ **Get enough physical exercise.** Yoga should do the trick!

- ✔ **Don't nap during the day.**

- ✔ **Avoid non-sleep activities (TV watching, reading, eating, and so on) in bed.**

- ✔ **Go to bed at the same time.** Make this a force of good habit.

- ✔ **Get up if you can't sleep and sit in another room.** Try going to bed again when you feel sleepy. Do this change of scenery as often as necessary instead of tormenting yourself in bed for hours on end.

- ✔ **Cut an hour off your regular eight-hour sleeping time.** Reducing your normal amount of sleep makes you that much more ready to sleep the next night.

We counsel against taking sleeping pills. They condition the body wrongly. If you feel that you need to take sleep aids, give herbal oils (massaged into the feet or the whole body), acupressure, or homeopathy a try. But many Yoga practitioners have found a significant improvement of their insomnia just after a few weeks of regular daily practice.

recruit your imagination for the purpose of falling soundly asleep? Here's how.

 If you're claustrophobic, this exercise may not necessarily work for you. But before giving up, you may first want to try evoking feelings of security and comfort, as in a mother's womb.

1. **Prepare yourself for sleep and lie down comfortably in bed in any position.**

2. **With closed eyes, breathe evenly through your nose for a while.**

3. **Now visualize yourself snugly enfolded in a protective cocoon of purple color.**

4. **While feeling safe in your purple environment, visualize a thin line of white light extending from the crown of your head to your solar plexus, just below your navel.**

This technique works even while traveling on a plane with the jets roaring next to your ears. Just tell the flight attendant not to disturb you while you're sleeping.

Yoga Nidra (Yogic Sleep)

If your body-mind is slow to wind down to get its well-deserved rest, here's a potent technique to catch up on your sleep quotient by enticing Mr. Sandman to visit you regularly. Yogic Sleep is a very powerful relaxation technique that you can do after you gain some control over the relaxation response (which we discuss in the earlier "Detach yourself" sidebar). When practiced successfully, this technique is as restorative as sleep — except you remain fully aware throughout.

To induce Yoga Nidra, you must listen to a set of instructions, similar to guided meditation. You can listen to a friend reading the instructions, but listening to a recording by someone else or by you yourself is more practical.

One feature of this practice is to focus in relatively quick succession on individual parts of the body. Mentally name each part and then sense it as distinctly as possible.

 In the beginning, you may find actually feeling certain body parts difficult. Don't let this setback dismay you; continue to rotate your awareness fairly swiftly. With practice, you can include in this circuit even the inner organs and all kinds of mental states.

Practicing Yoga Nidra before sleep is best because it's an excellent technique for inducing lucid dreaming and out-of-the-body experiences during sleep. *Lucid dreaming* refers to the kind of dream in which you're aware that you're dreaming. Great Yoga masters remain aware even during deep sleep. Only the body and brain are fast asleep, whereas awareness is continuous.

Formulating your intention

Yoga Nidra serves as a potent tool for reprogramming your brain. If you do it correctly, it can accelerate your inner or spiritual growth. It allows you to cultivate good habits and attitudes. First consider which specific habit or attitude you really want to replace with a more positive habit or attitude. This phase is called *formulating your intention.* Take your time to consider what you want to change about yourself.

Phrase your chosen intention in the following way: *I will become more this or that.* This wording affirms your life's future trajectory by enlisting the unconscious mind. Worthy intentions may be to become more patient, more tolerant, or more loving. We recommend that whatever intention you choose doesn't contradict any of Yoga's high moral virtues, which we discuss in Chapter 20. Also, make your intention realistic and specific. An intention like "I will become enlightened" is specific enough but perhaps not very realistic. By contrast, an intention like "I will become a better person" is too vague. A better intention is something more along the lines of "I will become more relaxed within myself," "I will become more tolerant toward others," or "I will become more patient." You want your intention to be something you can stick with until you realize it in your life rather than one you have to abandon because it was too lofty or undefined.

When formulating your intention, try to evoke the corresponding feeling inside you so you know what it feels like to be loving, patient, forgiving, or whatever.

After you set an intention, you formally apply it during the actual Yoga Nidra exercise (described in the following section) by repeating it when prompted.

Performing Yoga Nidra

The following steps show you how to perform Yoga Nidra:

1. **Choose a clear intention (as described in the preceding section) and lie flat on your back, with your arms stretched out by your sides (or whatever feels most comfortable).**

   Place a pillow or folded blanket behind your neck for support and another pillow or folded blanket under your knees for added comfort. Refer to Figure 4-1 earlier in the chapter.

2. **Close your eyes.**

3. **Repeat the clear intention you chose in Step 1 three times.**

4. **Take a couple of deep breaths, emphasizing exhalation.**

5. **Starting with your right side, rotate your awareness through all parts on that side of your body — limb by limb — in fairly quick succession.**

   Follow this progression: each finger, palm of the hand, back of the hand, the hand as a whole, forearm, elbow, upper arm, shoulder joint, shoulder, neck, each section of the face (forehead, eyes, nose, chin, and so on), ear, scalp, throat, chest, side of the rib cage, shoulder blade, waist, stomach, lower abdomen, genitals, buttocks, whole spine, thigh, top and back of knee, shin, calf, ankle, top of foot, heel, sole, each toe.

6. **Be aware of your body as a whole.**

7. **Repeat the rotation in Step 5 on the left side, ending with the whole-body awareness as described in Step 6.**

8. **Repeat Steps 5 through 7 one or more times until you achieve an adequate level of relaxation.**

9. **Continue to be aware of the whole body and the space surrounding it, feeling the stillness and peace.**

10. **Reaffirm your initial intention three times.**

11. **Mentally prepare to return to ordinary consciousness.**

12. **Gently move your fingers for a few moments, take a deep breath, and then open your eyes.**

No time limit applies to your Yoga Nidra performance, unless you impose one. Expect to come out of Yogic Sleep naturally, whether you return after only 15 minutes or a whole hour. Or you may just fall asleep. So if you have things to do afterward, make sure you set your wristwatch or clock for a gentle wake-up call. Don't rush up! Take your time to reintegrate with the ordinary world.

 I (Georg) swear by this practice. It's the most powerful yogic technique for personal change at the beginner level. Only the ecstatic state *(samadhi)* is more transformative. Several good recordings for practicing Yoga Nidra are available, but don't be surprised to discover that the instructions vary from recording to recording. For our choice, see the appendix.

Chapter 5

Breath and Movement Simplified

. . . .

In This Chapter

▶ Understanding breathing basics
▶ Detailing yogic breathing mechanics
▶ Linking breath and postural movement
▶ Adding sound to postural practice
▶ Introducing traditional methods of breath control

. . . .

The masters of Yoga discovered the usefulness of the breath thousands of years ago and in Hatha Yoga have perfected a system for the conscious control of breathing; in this chapter, we share their secrets with you. In the ancient Sanskrit language, the word for *breath* is the same as the word for *life* — *prana* (pronounced *prah-nah*) — which gives you a good clue about how important Yoga thinks breathing is for your well-being. Yoga without *prana* is like putting an empty pot on the stove and hoping for a delicious meal. In this chapter, we show you how to use conscious breathing in conjunction with the Yoga postures, and we also introduce several breathing exercises that you do seated either on a chair or in one of the Yoga sitting postures (if you're up to that).

Breathing Your Way to Good Health

Think of your breath as your most intimate friend. Your breath is with you from the moment you're born until you die. In a given day, you take between 20,000 and 30,000 breaths. Most likely, barring any respiratory problems, you're barely aware of your breathing. This state is akin to taking your best friend so for granted that the relationship gets stale and is put at risk. Although the automatic nature of breathing is part of the body's machinery that keeps you alive, having breathing occur automatically isn't necessarily to your advantage; automatic doesn't always mean optimal. In fact, most people's breathing habits are quite poor and to their great disadvantage. Stale air accumulates in their lungs and becomes as unproductive as a stale friendship. Poor breathing is known to cause and increase stress. Conversely, stress shortens your breath and increases your level of anxiety.

You can help alleviate stress through the simple practice of yogic breathing. Among other things, breathing loads your blood with oxygen, which, by nourishing and repairing your body's cells, maintains your health at the most desirable level. Shallow breathing, which is common, doesn't oxygenate the ten pints of blood circulating in your arteries and veins very efficiently. Consequently, toxins accumulate in the cells. Before you know it, you feel mentally sluggish and emotionally down, and eventually organs begin to malfunction. Is it any wonder that the breath is the best tool you have to profoundly affect your body and mind?

Bad breath is improved by brushing your teeth regularly and occasionally sucking on a mint. Bad breathing, however, is a bad habit that requires a bit more to change: You must retrain your body through breath awareness.

In Yoga, consciously regulated breathing has three major applications. Use it

✔ In conjunction with the various postures to achieve the deepest possible effect and to prepare the mind for meditation.

✔ As breath control (called *pranayama,* pronounced *prah-nah-yah-mah*) to invigorate your vitality.

✔ As a healing method in which you consciously direct the breath to a particular part or organ of the body to remove energetic blockages and facilitate healing. This practice is Yoga's gentle version of acupuncture.

Taking high-quality breaths

Before you jump right in and make drastic changes to your method of breathing, take a few minutes to assess your current breathing style. You may find it helpful to keep a log of your breathing habits over the course of a couple of days, noting how your breathing changes in accordance with the situations around you and your states of mind. Check your breathing by asking yourself the following questions:

✔ Is my breathing shallow (my abdomen and chest barely move when I fill my lungs with air)?

✔ Do I often breathe erratically (my breathing rhythm isn't harmonious)?

✔ Do I easily get out of breath?

120

✔ Is my breathing labored at times?

✔ Do I hold my breath in stressful situations?

✔ Do I generally breathe too fast?

If your answer to any of these questions is yes, you make an ideal candidate for yogic breathing. Even if you didn't answer yes, practicing conscious breathing still benefits your mind and body.

 Men take an average of 12 to 14 breaths per minute, and women take 14 to 15. Breathing at a markedly faster pace — usually associated with *chest breathing* — qualifies as hyperventilation, which leads to carbon dioxide depletion (your body needs some of this gas to maintain the right acid-alkaline balance of the blood).

The cosmic side of breathing

The Yoga scriptures state that humans take an average of 21,600 breaths per day. This number, which falls within the range accepted by modern research, is profoundly symbolic. Here's why: 21,600 is one-fifth of 108,000. The number 108, or multiples of it, is charged with special significance in India. The importance relates to the astronomical fact that the distance between the sun and the earth is 108 times greater than the sun's diameter. The symbolism is represented in the 108 beads of the rosary used by many Yoga practitioners in India. A full round on the rosary is a symbolic journey from the earth to heaven — that is, from ordinary consciousness to higher consciousness. And even the one-fifth is significant; 5 is the number associated with the air element. This correlation is one of many that Yoga masters profess between the human body-mind and the universe at large.

Relaxing with a couple of deep breaths

Think about the many times you've heard someone say "Now just take a couple of deep breaths and relax." This recommendation is so popular because it really works! Pain clinics across the country use breathing exercises for pain control. Childbirth preparation courses teach Yoga-related breathing techniques to both parents to aid the birthing process. Moreover, since the 1970s, stress gurus have taught yogic breathing to corporate America with great success.

Yogic breathing is like texting your nervous system with the message to relax. One easy way to experience the effect of simple breathing is to try the following exercise:

1. **Sit comfortably in your chair.**

2. **Close your eyes and visualize a swan gliding peacefully across a crystal-clear lake.**

3. **Now, like the swan, let your breath flow along in a long, smooth, and peaceful movement, ideally through your nose.**

   If your nose is plugged up, try to breathe through your nose and mouth, or just through your mouth.

4. **Extend your breath to its comfortable maximum for 20 rounds; then gradually let your breath return to normal.**

5. **Afterward, take a few moments to sit with your eyes closed and notice the difference in how you feel overall.**

   Can you imagine how relaxed and calm you'd feel after 10 to 15 minutes of conscious yogic breathing?

Practicing safe yogic breathing

As you look forward to the calming and restorative power of yogic breathing, take time to reflect on a few safety tips that can help you enjoy your experience.

- If you have problems with your lungs (such as a cold or asthma), or if you have a heart disease, consult your physician first before embarking on breath control even under the supervision of a Yoga therapist (unless he or she happens to be a physician as well).

- Don't practice breathing exercises when the air is too cold or too hot.

- Avoid practicing in polluted air, including the smoke from incense. Whenever possible, practice breath control outdoors or with an open window, where you maximize exposure to *negative ions* (atoms with a negative electronic charge). Negative ions in moderation are considered beneficial for health. On the other hand, positive ions, which are produced by your TV and computer, have been connected with fatigue, headaches, and respiratory problems.

- Don't strain your breathing — remain relaxed while doing the breathing exercises.

- Don't overdo the number of repetitions. Stay within our guidelines for each exercise.

- Don't wear any constricting pants or belts.

Reaping the benefits of yogic breathing

In addition to relaxing the body and calming the mind, yogic breathing offers an entire spectrum of other benefits that work like insurance, protecting your investment in a longer and healthier life. Here are six important advantages of controlled breathing:

- It steps up your metabolism (which helps with weight control).

- It uses muscles that automatically help improve your posture, preventing the stiff, slumped carriage characteristic of many older people.

- It keeps the lung tissue elastic, which allows you to take in more oxygen to nourish the 50 trillion cells in your body.

- It tones your abdominal area, a common site for health problems because many illnesses begin in the intestines.

- It helps strengthen your immune system.

- It reduces your levels of tension and anxiety.

Breathing through your nose (most of the time)

No matter what anybody else tells you, yogic breathing typically occurs through the nose, both during inhalation and exhalation. For traditional yogis and yoginis, the mouth is meant for eating and the nose for breathing. We know at least three good reasons for breathing through the nose:

- It slows down the breath because you're breathing through two small openings rather than the one big opening in your mouth, and slow is good in Yoga.

- The air is hygienically filtered and warmed by the nasal passages. Even the purest air contains, at the

Real-life stories on the benefits of yogic breathing

The late T. Krishnamacharya of Chennai (Madras), India — one of the great Yoga masters of the 20th century — is a classic illustration of the benefits of yogic breathing. On his 100th birthday celebration, he initiated the ceremony by chanting a 30-second-long continuous *om* sound. He also sat up perfectly straight on the floor for many hours every day during the festivities, which lasted several days. Not bad for a centenarian!

To give another example, Chris Briscoe is a baby-boomer beauty, the mother of two grown boys, and a long-time popular resident and community leader in Malibu, California. In her 20s, she developed asthma and for 25 years was on heavy medication and allergy shots. If Chris woke up in the morning wheezing, she could count on being in the hospital by that evening. Aerobic exercise and allergies also induced her asthma. In 1990, Chris attended her first Yoga class with me (Larry) at the Malibu Community Center, where she learned yogic breathing and the principles of breath and movement. After only three months of attending classes twice a week, practicing yogic breathing at home, and taking Chinese herbs, Chris was able to stop taking her asthma medication and allergy shots. She has remained in class and off medication almost entirely for the past 19 years. ***Note:*** We must stress, however, that you consult with your physician before discontinuing prescribed medication.

least, dust particles and, at the worst, all the toxic pollutants of a metropolis.

✔ According to traditional Yoga, nasal breathing stimulates the subtle energy center — the so-called *ajna-cakra* (pronounced *ah-gyah-chuk-rah*) located near sinuses in the spot between the eyebrows. This very important location is the meeting place of the left (cooling) and the right (heating) current of vital energy *(prana)* that act directly on the nervous and endocrine systems. (For the two currents, see the "Alternate nostril breathing" section later in this chapter.)

Folk wisdom teaches that every rule has its exception, which is definitely the case with the yogic rule of breathing through the nose. A few classical yogic techniques for breath control require you to breathe through the mouth. When we present a mouth-breathing technique, we alert you to that fact.

What if I can't breathe through my nose?

Some folks suffer from various physiological conditions that prevent them from breathing through their noses. Of course, Yoga is flexible. If you have difficulty breathing when lying down, try sitting up. The time of day can also make a difference in your ability to breathe. For example, you may be more congested or exposed to more allergens in the morning than in the afternoon. You, of course, can detect the differences.

If you're still not sure how to settle on a comfortable breathing method, first try inhaling through your nose and exhaling through your mouth and, failing this, just breathe through your mouth and don't worry for now. Worry is always counterproductive.

How about breathing through my nose all the time?

Many Americans participate in more than one kind of physical activity or exercise discipline. Each has its own guidelines and rules for breathing, which we suggest you follow. For example, the majority of aerobic activities —

running, walking, weight lifting, and so on — recommend that you inhale through the nose and exhale through the mouth. The reason: You need to move a lot of air quickly in and out of your lungs. And breathing only through the nose while swimming can be very dangerous. In fact, we don't recommend underwater *pranayama* unless you enjoy a snootful of water making its way to your lungs.

 In the beginning, save yogic breathing for your Yoga exercises. Later, when you become more skillful at it, you may want to adopt nasal breathing during all normal activities. You can then benefit from its calming and hygienic effects throughout the day.

Notice your breath

When you pay close attention to the rhythm of your breath, you may be surprised to notice that it has several parts. According to Yoga, the four aspects of controlled breathing are:

- Inhalation *(puraka,* pronounced *poo-rah-kah)*

- Retention or holding after inhalation *(antar-kumbhaka,* pronounced *ahn-tahr-koom-bhah-kah)*

- Exhalation *(recaka,* pronounced *reh-chah-kah)*

- Retention or holding after exhalation *(bahya-kumbhaka,* pronounced *bah-yah-koom-bhah-kah)*

In this book, we emphasize exhalation. Some classical Yoga authorities also refer to a type of retention that occurs spontaneously and effortlessly in some higher states of consciousness. This retention is known as *kevala-kumbhaka* (pronounced *keh-vah-lah-koom-bhah-kah),* or absolute retention.

127

The Mechanics of Yogic Breathing

Most people are either shallow chest breathers or shallow belly breathers. Yogic breathing incorporates a complete breath that expands both the chest and the abdomen on inhalation either from the chest down or the abdomen up. Both are valid techniques. (Figures 5-2 and 5-3 later in the chapter show you each of these techniques.)

Yogic breathing involves breathing much more deeply than usual, which in turn brings more oxygen into your system. Don't be surprised if you feel a little lightheaded or even dizzy in the beginning. If this situation happens during your Yoga practice, just rest for a few minutes or lie down until you feel like proceeding. Remind yourself that you don't need to rush.

Some Yoga practitioners think that you can breathe into parts of the body other than the lungs. Not so. You inhale the breath through either your nose or mouth, and it then expands into the lungs. You may perceive that the breath is moving up and down throughout the body, but you're actually feeling muscle contraction. Any suggestion of an up or down movement of the breath is due entirely to the sequence of your muscular control and the flow of your attention.

In both chest and abdominal breathing, the abdomen draws in on exhalation. From a mechanical standpoint, Yogic breathing moves the spine and works the muscles and organs of respiration, which primarily include the diaphragm, *intercostal* (between the ribs) and abdominal muscles, and the lungs and heart. The diaphragm pulls down when it contracts, which creates more space for the lungs during inhalation. The chest noticeably widens. When the diaphragm relaxes it moves back into its upward curve, forcing the air out of the lungs.

The *diaphragm* is a vaulted muscle sheath that separates the lungs and heart from the stomach, liver, kidneys, and other abdominal organs. It's attached all around the lower border of the rib cage and, by a pair of powerful muscles, to the first through fourth lumbar vertebrae. The diaphragm and the chest muscles activate the lungs, which don't have muscles.

Understanding how your emotions affect your diaphragm

Psychologically, people tend to use the diaphragm as a lid to bottle up their undigested or unwanted emotions of anger and fear. Chronic contraction of the diaphragm makes it inflexible and blocks the free flow of energy between the abdomen (the nether region of the bowels) and the chest (the feelings associated with the heart). Yogic breathing helps restore flexibility and function to the diaphragm and removes obstructions to the flow of physical and emotional energy. You can then experience liberation of your emotions, which can lead you to integrate them with the rest of your life.

Deep breathing not only affects the organs in your chest and abdomen but also reaches down into your gut emotions. Don't be surprised if sighs and perhaps even a few tears accompany the tension release your breath work achieves. These are welcome signs that you're peeling off the muscular armor you have placed around your abdomen and heart. Instead of feeling concerned or embarrassed, rejoice in your newly gained inner freedom! Yoga practitioners know that real men do cry.

Appreciating the complete yogic breath

If shallow or erratic breathing puts your well-being at risk, the complete yogic breath is your ticket to excellent physical and mental health. If you do no other Yoga exercise, the complete Yoga breath — integrally combined with relaxation — can still be of invaluable benefit to you. It's your secret weapon, except Yoga doesn't advocate the use of force.

Belly breathing

Before you jump into practicing the complete yogic breath, try out this exercise:

1. **Lie flat on your back and place one hand on your chest and the other on your abdomen as in Figure 5-1.**

   Place a small pillow or folded blanket under your head if you have tension in your neck or if your chin tilts upward. Place a large pillow under your knees if your back is uncomfortable.

Figure 5-1:
Your hand position helps you detect motion during belly breathing.

2. **Take 15 to 20 slow, deep breaths.**

   During inhalation, expand your abdomen; during

exhalation, contract your abdomen but keep your chest as motionless as possible. Your hands act as motion detectors.

3. **Pause for a couple of seconds between inhalation and exhalation keeping the throat soft.**

Belly-to-chest breathing

In belly-to-chest breathing, you really exercise your chest and diaphragm muscles as well as your lungs and treat your body with oodles of oxygen and life force *(prana)*. When you're done, your cells are humming with energy, and your brain is very grateful to you for the extra boost. You can use this form of breathing before you begin your relaxation practice, before and where indicated during your practice of the Yoga postures, and in fact whenever you feel so inclined throughout the day. You don't necessarily have to lie down as we describe in the following exercise. You can be seated or even walking. After practicing this technique for a while, you may find that it becomes second nature to you.

1. **Lie flat on your back, with your knees bent and your feet on the floor at hip width, and relax.**

   Place a small pillow or folded blanket under your head if you have tension in your neck or if your chin tilts upward. Place a large pillow under your knees if your back is uncomfortable.

2. **Inhale while expanding your abdomen, your ribs and then your chest.**

   Pause for a couple of seconds.

Figure 5-2:
The classic Yoga breath.

3. **Exhale while releasing your chest and shoulder muscles, gently and continuously contracting or drawing your abdomen in as shown in Figure 5-2.**

   Pause again for a couple of seconds.

4. **Repeat Steps 2 and 3 six to twelve times.**

You can greatly enhance the value of this and other exercises by fully participating with your mind. Feel the air fill your lungs. Feel your muscles work. Feel your body as a whole. Visualize precious life energy entering your lungs and every cell of your body, rejuvenating and energizing you. To help you experience this exercise more profoundly, keep your eyes closed. Place your hands on your abdomen and feel it expand upon inhalation.

Chest-to-belly breathing

Classically, yoga teachers taught yogic breathing from the abdomen up on inhalation (see the preceding section), which you can see in numerous publications on Yoga. This method works very well for many people. However, in the 1960s, Yoga master T.K.V. Desikachar, with the guidance of his father, the late T. Krishnamacharya, began to adapt the traditional yogic breathing to the needs of their Western students. Think about it! Folks in the West sit in chairs and bend forward too much. The daily sitting routine begins in the early morning when they go to the bathroom and then lean over the sink to brush their teeth and do whatever else

132

they do to their faces. They sit at the breakfast table and then again while they commute to their workplaces, where they clock a lot more time sitting and slouching in front of a computer or typewriter or bending over a machine. Finally, in the evening, they go come home and sit down for dinner and afterward, perhaps, sit in front of the television or their computer until their eyes get blurry.

The chest-to-belly breathing emphasizes arching the spine and the upper back to compensate for all this bending forward throughout the day, and it also works very well for moving in and out of Yoga postures. Chest-to-belly breathing is also an excellent energizer in the morning; you can even do it before you hop out of bed. We don't recommend this exercise late at night, though, because it's likely to keep you awake.

The following exercise complements the belly-to-chest breathing we cover in the preceding section. As with that technique, you can practice the following exercise lying down, seated, or even while walking.

1. **Lie flat on your back, with your knees bent and the feet on the floor at hip width, and relax.**

   Place a small pillow or folded blanket under your head if you have tension in your neck or if your chin tilts upward. Place a large pillow under your knees if your back is uncomfortable.

2. **Inhale while expanding the chest from the top down and continuing this movement downward into the belly as shown in Figure 5-3a.**

   Pause for a couple of seconds.

Figure 5-3:
The new Yoga breath.

3. **Exhale while gently contracting and drawing the belly inward, starting just below the navel as in Figure 5-3b.**

   Pause for a couple of seconds.

4. **Repeat Steps 2 and 3 six to twelve times.**

Starting out with focus breathing

If you have a little difficulty synchronizing yourself with the rhythm of the complete Yoga breathing techniques, you may want to try a simpler method we call *focus breathing* first. Focus breathing is a great stepping stone to all the other techniques. The following list walks you through the phases of focus breathing:

- **Phase one:** During your Yoga practice, simply follow the directions we give you about when to inhale and exhale for each posture, breathe only through the nose, and make the breath a little longer than normal. That's all you have to do! Don't worry about where the breath is starting or ending, just breathe slowly and evenly. (We present the postures in Part II.)

- **Phase two:** After you're used to the phase-one practice, just add a short pause of one or two seconds after inhalation and another one after exhalation.

✔ **Phase three:** When you're comfortable with the practices of phases one and two, add drawing the belly in during exhalation without force or exaggeration.

Realizing the power of a pause

During your normal shallow breathing, you notice a slight natural pause between inhalation and exhalation. This pause becomes very important in yogic breathing; even though it only lasts one or two seconds, the pause is a natural moment of stillness and meditation. If you pay attention to this pause, it can help you become more aware of the unity between body, breath, and mind — all of which are key elements in your Yoga practice. With the help of a teacher, you also can discover how to lengthen the pause during various Yoga postures to heighten its positive effects.

Partners in Yoga: Breath and Postural Movement

In Hatha Yoga, breathing is just as important as the postures, which we describe in Part II. How you breathe when you're moving into, holding, or moving out of any given posture can greatly increase the efficiency and the benefits of your practice. Think of the breath as mileage plus. The more you use breathing consciously, the more mileage you gain for your health and longevity. Here are some basic guidelines:

✔ **Let the breath surround the movement.** The breath leads the movement by a couple of moments; that is, you initiate breathing (both inhalation and exhalation), and then you make the movement. When you inhale, the body opens or expands, and when you exhale, the body folds or contracts.

✔ **Both the inhalation and the exhalation end with a natural pause.**

✔ **In the beginning, let the breath dictate the length of the postural movement.** For example, if you're raising your arms as you inhale and you run out of breath before you reach your goal, just pause your breathing for a moment and then bring your arms back down as you exhale. With practice, your breath gradually gets longer.

✔ **Let the breath itself be your teacher.** When your breath sounds labored, you need to back off or come out of a posture.

✔ **Try to visualize the breath flowing into the area you're working with any given posture.**

Breathing in four directions

You can move your body in four natural directions:

✔ **Flexion:** Bending forward

✔ **Extension:** Bending backward

✔ **Lateral flexion:** Bending sideways

✔ **Rotation:** Twisting your body

Normally, when people move they tend to hold or strain their breath. In Yoga, you simply follow the natural flow of the breath. As a rule, adopt this pattern:

✔ Inhale when moving into back bends (as shown in Figure 5-4a).

- ✔ Exhale when moving into forward bends (see Figure 5-4b).

- ✔ Exhale when moving into side bends (see Figure 5-4c).

- ✔ Exhale when moving into twists (as shown in Figure 5-4d).

Figure 5-4: Breathing properly during postures is important.

Recognizing the distinct roles of movement and holding in Yoga postures

Most Yoga books talk about *stationary* or *held* Yoga postures *(asanas)*. We suggest that before trying to hold a posture, you first become acquainted with moving in and out of most of the postures we recommend in this book, following the rules of breath and movement in the preceding section. When you can move in and out of a given posture easily and confidently, try holding the posture for a short period *without* holding or straining your breath. You know you're straining when your face turns into a grimace or you feel it going red like a tomato. Getting a handle on moving into and out of the postures before adding the element of holding is important for three reasons:

- ✔ It helps prepare your muscles and joints by bringing circulation to the area. It's like juicing up your joints, which adds a safety factor.

- ✔ It helps you experience the intimate connection between body, breath, and mind.

- ✔ In the case of stretching postures, moving in and out of a given posture before holding the posture supports the concept of *Proprioceptive Neuromuscular Facilitation* (PNF). If you tighten a muscle before stretching it either by gentle resistance *(isotonic)* or by pushing against a fixed force *(isometric),* the subsequent stretch is deeper than just using a static pose. Scientific research supports this phenomenon; numerous physical therapy texts refer to it as PNF.

The Yoga Miracle

To see and experience firsthand the power of PNF (introduced in the preceding section) in the context of Yoga, grab yourself a partner and follow these instructions for what we call The Yoga Miracle. You find that you can achieve a deeper stretch than you normally would.

1. **Lie on your back, with your left leg bent and your left foot on the floor; your right leg is up in the air and slightly bent.**

   Ask your partner to kneel in the lunge position near your feet.

2. **Have your partner test the flexibility of your hamstrings by holding the back of your right**

heel and pushing it gently towards you until you reach the first resistance point.

The partner on the floor is relaxed and doesn't resist. (See Figure 5-5a.) Be sure not to force anything.

3. **Bring your right leg back to the starting point and then begin to push against the kneeling partner's hand as shown in Figure 5-5b.**

The kneeling partner now either gently resists your right foot completely (isometrically) or allows your foot to move a little with resistance (isotonically).

Both tests produce the same effect. As you push against your partner's hand, your right hamstring muscles tighten. You want these muscles to tighten for about ten seconds.

Figure 5-5:
Test your new flexibility and behold the Yoga Miracle.

4. **After approximately ten seconds, the partner on the ground relaxes the right leg and then allows the standing partner to repeat Step 2 (see Figure 5-5c).**

   Compare the results to those from the original Step 2 stretch and behold the Yoga Miracle!

 Don't try to push your partner over, just push until you feel your leg muscles tighten. Next, after about ten seconds, release your leg and allow your partner to stretch you again by gently pushing against your heel, causing your leg to move toward you in a stretch that's not forced, as shown in Figure 5-5c. See how far you can extend this time. You may be pleasantly surprised!

Answering common breath and movement questions

Getting the hang of breath and movement takes a bit of work when you tackle them separately, and combining them successfully can be even trickier. The following sections give you some tips on handling both.

How much should I move and how long should I hold?

We note the number of repetitions and how long to hold them in all our recommended programs. With practice, you develop an idea of what's right for you; a lot depends on how you feel at any given moment. In general, we suggest at least three but no more than eight repetitions for a *dynamic,* or moving, posture. You can put together a program that has only moving postures, but normally we recommend a combination of both *static* (still) and dynamic postures.

We often ask you to hold a posture for six to eight breaths, which translates to roughly 30 seconds. Keep breathing when you hold a posture — don't hold your breath.

What about bouncing when I hold a stretching posture?

Now and then, we still see eager Yoga practitioners seeking to achieve better flexibility by bouncing during the holding phase of a stretching posture. This practice is part of old-school training, which really isn't such a good habit after all. Bouncing not only tends to disconnect you from the breath but also can be risky, especially if your muscles are stiff or not adequately warmed up. Be kind to yourself!

How do I start combining breath with movement?

The arrows in the following exercise and wherever they appear in this book tell you the direction of postural movement and the part of the breath that goes with the movement. *Inhale* means inhalation, *exhale* means exhalation, and *breaths* means the number of breaths defining the length of a postural hold.

1. **Lie on your back comfortably with your legs straight or bent.**

   Place your arms at your sides near your hips with your palms turned down (see Figure 5-6a).

2. **Inhale through your nose and, after one or two seconds, begin to slowly raise your arms up over your head — in sync with inhalation — until they touch the ground behind you (see Figure 5-6b).**

   Leave your arms slightly bent.

3. **When you reach the end of inhalation, pause**

141

for one or two seconds even if your arms don't make it to the floor and then exhale slowly through your nose and bring your arms back to your sides along the same path.

Figure 5-6:
The breath surrounds the movement.

4. **Repeat Steps 2 and 3 with a nice slow rhythm.**

   Remember, open or expand as you inhale, fold or contract as you exhale.

After you become comfortable with this exercise, combine it with our recommended breathing techniques from earlier in this chapter: focus breathing (which we cover in "Starting out with Focus Breathing") or any of the techniques in "Appreciating the complete yogic breath" (belly breathing, belly-to-chest breathing, or chest-to-belly breathing). You can decide which technique you prefer as you begin combining breathing with movement.

Sounding Off: Yogic Breathing

Sound, which is a form of vibration, is one of the means that Yoga employs to harmonize the vibration of your body and mind. In fact, the repetition of special sounds is one of the older and more potent techniques of Yoga. Here, we show you how to try this technique in conjunction with conscious breathing. A good way to start is to use the soft-sounding syllables *ah, ma,* and *sa.* (We're not asking you to chant, although chanting can be a great and useful experi-

142

ence as well.) Sound makes your exhalation longer and also tightens your abdominal muscles.

Try the following exercise while sitting in a chair or on the floor:

1. **Take a deep breath, and then as you exhale make a long _ah_ sound in a way that you find pleasing and comfortable.**

   Continue the same sound for as long as your exhalation lasts. Then take a resting breath in between and repeat the exercise a total of five times.

2. **Relax for a few moments and next do five repetitions with the sound _ma_.**

Good vibes

Yoga masters have long known that the universe is an ocean of vibrations. Some have maintained that even the ultimate reality is a state of continuous vibration — but a vibration that exceeds the three dimensions of space. Some quantum physicists call this entity a _holomovement._ The Sanskrit word for vibration is _spanda_ (pronounced _spun-dah_). According to Yoga, the human body and mind are constantly vibrating. However, this vibration is more or less disharmonious and out of sync with the super-vibration of the _ultimate reality_ (which we cover in Chapters 1 and 21). This disharmony creates unhappiness, alienation, and a sense of being separate from the physical world. The purpose of Yoga is to remove this disharmony and synchronize the body and mind with the ultimate reality, restoring joy and the sense of being connected with everyone and everything.

3. Relax again and conclude by using the sound *sa* five times.

After you complete the full cycle, just sit quietly for a few minutes and notice how relaxed you feel.

True yogic breathing also includes the *throat sound,* which forms part of the traditional practice of *ujjayi* (pronounced *ooh-jah-yee*), or "victorious" breath control. This more advanced technique is often mistakenly identified as sound breathing. The *ujjayi* sound is produced with the mouth closed and by breathing through the nose. By slightly constricting the throat during inhalation and exhalation, you produce a soft hissing sound similar to a baby's breathing or a very gentle snore. This technique is easiest to pick up during exhalation; you can then gradually apply it to the inhalation phase. If you're making the sound properly, you notice a slight contraction of your abdomen. You want your exhale to be audible to you but not to someone standing four feet away from you. Certainly don't strain to the point where you make a grimace! If the throat sound doesn't happen for you right away, just leave it until later — no need to rush.

This kind of breathing stimulates the energetic center at the throat and is quite relaxing. Some evidence states that it slows down the heart rate, lowers blood pressure, and induces a deeper and more restful sleep.

Practicing Breath Control the Traditional Way

Hatha Yoga includes various methods of breath control, all of which belong to the more advanced practices and traditionally follow extensive purification of body and mind.

Some Western teachers have incorporated these methods into their beginner's classes, but our experience shows us that they're best at the intermediary to advanced levels. There are, however, three methods that we believe are suitable for beginners if you practice them with the necessary modifications and precautions.

Traditional Hatha Yoga emphasizes holding the breath — not a good idea for beginners. In this section, we focus on techniques that are safe for any healthy person to practice.

 The cooling methods discussed in this section are best done in warm weather to avoid overcooling.

Alternate nostril breathing

Lab researchers have demonstrated what Yoga masters have known for hundreds, if not thousands, of years: Humans don't breathe evenly through both nostrils. In a two-to-three-hour cycle, the nostrils become alternately dominant. It appears that left-nostril breathing is particularly connected with functions of the left cerebral hemisphere (notably verbal skills), and right-nostril breathing seems to connect more with the right hemisphere (notably spatial performance).

The technique called *alternate nostril breathing* goes by various others names, including *nadi-shodhana* ("channel cleansing," pronounced *nah-dee-shod-hah-nah*). The following steps help you tackle it at the beginning level:

1. **Sit comfortably on a chair or in one of the yogic sitting postures with your back straight (see Chapter 7).**

2. **Check which nostril has the most air flowing through it and begin alternative breathing with the open nostril.**

Expanding the life force through Yoga

According to Yoga, the breath is just the material aspect of an energy that is far more subtle and universal. Called *prana* (pronounced *prah-nah*), which means both "breath" and "life," this energy corresponds to the Chinese concept *chi,* known to a growing number of Westerners from acupuncture and Far Eastern martial arts.

This life force underlies everything that exists and, ultimately, is the power *(shakti,* pronounced *shuk-tee)* aspect of the spirit itself. When *prana* leaves the body, a person dies. Thus, the practitioners of Hatha Yoga seek to carefully preserve the life force and enhance or expand it as much as possible. The most significant practice for doing so is *pranayama* (pronounced *prah-nah-yah-mah*), a Sanskrit term that is often incorrectly explained as being composed of *prana* and *yama* ("control"). In fact, it drives from *prana* and *ayama* (pronounced *ah-yah-mah*) — the expansion or extension of the life force. So, although the term is conveniently translated as "breath control," it's actually much more.

Science has solved many mysteries but is still puzzled about life itself. Some scientists now believe that a subtle, vital energy that can't be reduced to biochemistry does indeed operate in the body. They have named it *bioenergy* or *bioplasma*. Through Yoga, especially yogic breathing, you can come to control that energy, whatever you want to call it, in your own body. Some Yoga masters can even influence the life force in someone else's body, helping them to heal or speeding up their spiritual awakening.

If both are equally open, all the better. In that case, begin with the left nostril.

You can check which nostril is dominant simply by breathing through one nostril and then the other and comparing the two flows.

3. **Place your right hand so that your thumb is on the right nostril and the little and ring fingers are on the left nostril, with the index and middle fingers tucked against the ball of the thumb.**

   Note: According to some authorities, you should place the index and middle fingers on the spot between the eyebrows (known as the *third eye*). We recommend the other method if it feels comfortable to you.

4. **Close the blocked nostril and, mentally counting to five, inhale gently but fully through the open nostril — don't strain (see Figure 5-7).**

5. **Open the blocked nostril and close the other nostril and exhale, again mentally counting to five.**

6. **Inhale through the same nostril to the count of five, and exhale through the opposite nostril, repeating 10 to 15 times.**

As your lung capacity improves, you can make your inhalations and exhalations longer, but *never* force the breath. Gradually increase the overall duration of the exercise from, say, 3 minutes to 15 minutes.

Figure 5-7:
Alternate nostril breathing.

The cooling breath

This technique, which in Sanskrit is called *shitali* (pronounced *sheet-ah-lee*), gets its name from the cooling effect that it has on the body and the mind. Traditionally, the cooling breath is believed to remove fever, still hunger, quench thirst, and alleviate diseases of the spleen. Here's how you practice it:

1. **Sit in a comfortable Yoga posture or on a chair and relax your body.**

2. **Curl your tongue lengthwise and let its tip protrude from your mouth as shown in Figure 5-8.**

Figure 5-8:
Curled tongue for cooling breath.

3. **Slowly suck in air through the tube formed by your tongue and exhale gently through the nose**

   Repeat this breath 10 to 15 times.

If you can't curl your tongue — which is a genetic ability — you can practice the Crow's Beak instead. This technique is technically known as *kaki-mudra* ("crow's gesture," pronounced *kah-kee-moo-drah*). Here you pucker your mouth, leaving just a small space for the air to pass through. Inhale through the mouth and exhale through the nose as with *shitali*.

Shitkari: Inhaling through the mouth

Shitkari (pronounced *sheet-kah-ree*) is another technique that calls for inhalation through the mouth, and its effects are similar to the cooling breath we discuss in the preceding section. The term means "that which makes a sucking sound." Sitting upright and relaxed, move through the following routine:

1. **Open your mouth but keep your teeth closed, as if you were going to brush your front teeth.**

2. **Place the tip of the tongue against the palate behind the upper teeth.**

   Keep your eyes closed and make sure that you don't squint your face.

3. **Inhale through your teeth and breathe out through your nose.**

   Repeat the inhalation and exhalation 10 to 15 times.

TIP

If your gums are sensitive or a visit to the dentist is long overdue, avoid doing this practice when the air is cool.

Kapala-bhati: Frontal sinus cleansing

Kapala-bhati (pronounced *kah-pah-la-bhah-tee*) literally means "skull luster" and is also known as *frontal sinus* (or *brain) cleansing*. The curious Sanskrit name is explained by the fact that the technique causes a sense of luminosity in the head, as well as lightheadedness, especially when you're overdoing it. Sometimes this breathing method is wrongly equated with *bhastrika* ("bellows"), which is a more advanced technique of rapid breathing, but *kapala-bhati* belongs to the preparatory practices of traditional Hatha Yoga. The technique requires rapid inhalation and exhalation through the nose with short staccato breaths, with emphasis on exhalation.

Kapala-bhati is a very energizing technique that you can use to combat physical or mental fatigue, so if you value your sleep, don't practice it at night. It can also warm your body (but be careful to avoid practicing this technique in cold air!). Before attempting the following exercise, get the hang of relaxing your abdomen during inhalation and pulling it in during exhalation. Gradually shorten the exhalations.

1. **Sit, if you can, in a comfortable cross-legged**

posture, holding your spine straight and resting your hands in your lap.

2. **Take a few deep breaths and, after your last inhalation, do 15 to 20 fast exhalations each followed by a short inhalation, using the nose to inhale and exhale.**

   Repeat this step twice. With each exhalation, which lasts only for half a second, pull in your abdomen.

If you're contracting your facial or shoulder muscles during *kapala-bhati,* you're not practicing correctly. Remember to stay relaxed and let the abdominal muscles do most of the work.

I've got the whole world in my breath

According to Yoga, everyone is interconnected and part of the same single reality. You can make this abstract fact more concrete and personal when you consider the breath. Each breath you take contains about ten sextillion atoms, which is the number 1 followed by 22 zeros. Multiply this by 6 billion people and by roughly 21,000 exhalations per day. Every time you take a breath, you inhale an average of one atom from the exhaled atoms in the atmosphere. Upon exhalation, you contribute to the collective store of exhaled breaths. Therefore, you're literally sharing other people's breaths and life energies, and they are sharing yours.

Part II

Postures for Health Maintenance and Restoration

The 5th Wave By Rich Tennant

@RICHTENNANT

"This position is good for reaching inner calm, mental clarity, and things that roll behind the refrigerator."

In this part . . .

This part is, as they say, where the action is. These chapters build on the ideas in Part I, so if you're not familiar with those concepts, we suggest you hit Part I before proceeding.

Here we introduce dozens of Hatha Yoga postures for a balanced and varied exercise program. For your convenience, we organize the Yoga postures into basic categories, such as sitting, standing, bending, twisting, balancing, inverted, and dynamic postures. Finally, we guide you through a sample beginners' routine to help you get started.

Chapter 6

Please Be Seated

● ●

In This Chapter
▶ Discovering the traditional purpose and benefits of postures
▶ Starting out slow and safe with easier postures

● ●

Culture greatly influences the way humans sit. People in the Eastern hemisphere favor squatting on their haunches or sitting cross-legged on the floor, but most Westerners are only comfortable sitting on chairs — as you're probably doing right now as you read this book. Actually, your everyday sitting preferences have a decided effect on your capacity to feel steady and comfortable in the Yoga postures, whether standing or sitting.

If you're new to Yoga and its sitting postures, you'll soon discover that a lifetime of chair-sitting exacts a stiff price. Your work with the postures in this book can help you gradually improve your floor sitting, but until you're ready to make the transition to the floor, use a chair when you sit for formal practice. After all, two of the larger Yoga organizations in the world, The Self-Realization Fellowship

(SRF) and Transcendental Meditation (TM), encourage their Western practitioners to use a chair for meditation and breathing exercises.

In this chapter, we describe the following sitting postures that you can use for relaxation, meditation, breath control, various cleansing practices, or as a starting point for other postures:

- ✔ Chair-sitting posture
- ✔ Easy posture
- ✔ Thunderbolt posture
- ✔ Auspicious posture
- ✔ Perfect posture

 Many other sitting postures exist in Yoga; you can gradually add to your basic repertoire as your joints become more flexible and your back muscles gain strength.

Understanding the Philosophy of Yoga Postures

Postures, or *asanas* (pronounced *ah-sah-nahs*) in Sanskrit, are probably the part of Yoga that you're most familiar with. They're those poses that look impossible but that are done with ease by many Yoga students. Beyond stretching and increasing strength and flexibility, Yoga postures help you get in tune with yourself, your body, and your environment. Through *asanas,* you can begin to see yourself as one with your environment.

 For traditional Yoga masters, *asanas* are just one part of the yogic system. Postures are the basis of the third limb of the classical eightfold path of Yoga formulated by Yoga master Patanjali. (Flip to Chapter 20 for more on the eight-fold path.)

Yogic postures are more than mere bodily poses — they're also expressions of your state of mind. An *asana* is poise, composure, carriage — all words suggesting an element of balance and refinement. The postures demonstrate the profound connection between body and mind.

Traditional Yoga experts view the body as a temple dedicated to the spirit. They believe that you must keep the body pure and beautiful to honor the spiritual reality it houses. Each posture is another way of remembering that higher principle — commonly called the *spirit, divine,* or *transcendental Self* — that the body enshrines. If you prefer to practice Yoga without such ideas, you can still use posture as a way of connecting with nature at large because your body isn't totally isolated from its environment. Where exactly does your body end, and where exactly does the surrounding space begin? How much does your body's electromagnetic field extend beyond your skin? How far away did the oxygen particles that are now part of your body originate?

According to traditional Yoga manuals, the main purpose of *asana* is to prepare the body to sit quietly, easily, and steadily for breathing exercises and meditation. The way you sit is an important foundation technique for these practices; when you perform them properly, the sitting postures act as natural "tranquilizers" for the body, and when the physical vehicle is still, the mind soon follows.

If your knees are more than a few inches higher than your hips when you sit cross-legged on the floor, it's an indication that your hip joints are tight. If you try to sit for a long while in this position for meditation or breathing exercises, you may very well end up with an aching back. Don't feel

Asana by any other name

The term *asana* simply means "sitting." It can denote both the surface you sit on and the bodily posture. An alternative term is *tirtha,* or "pilgrimage center," which suggests that practitioners shouldn't approach Yoga postures casually but respectfully, with great mental focus.

Some postures are called *mudras* (pronounced *moo-drahs*) or "seals," because they're especially effective in keeping the life energy *(prana)* sealed within the body. This leads to greater vitality and better mental focusing. Life energy is everywhere, both inside and outside the body, but you must properly harness it within the body in order to promote health and happiness.

bad — you're not alone. Accept your current limitations in this area and use a prop, like a firm cushion or thickly folded blanket, to raise your buttocks off the floor high enough to drop your knees at least level with your hips.

 If you attend a lecture or other special gathering at a Hatha Yoga center, remember that few, if any, chairs are usually available, so be prepared to sit on the floor. If you aren't accustomed to sitting cross-legged on the floor with an unsupported back, bring along a prop, such as a firm cushion or a blanket, to raise your buttocks (see Chapter 19). Arrive early so that you can find a wall or post to sit against to support your back. If none of these ideas sits well with you (no pun intended), just bring your own folding chair and sit near the rear of the room.

Looking at the Many Variations of Sitting

Some contemporary Hatha Yoga manuals feature more than 50 sitting postures, which demonstrate not only the inventiveness of Yoga practitioners but also the body's amazing versatility. Yet, all you may ever need or want are perhaps half a dozen yogic sitting postures. The following sections describe some good sitting postures and show you how to execute them.

 For postures that involve sitting on the floor, raising your buttocks off the floor on a firm cushion or thickly folded blanket is helpful because it allows you to sit comfortably and stably without slumping.

Be sure to alternate the cross of the legs from day to day when practicing any of the sitting postures because you don't want to become lopsided.

Chair-sitting posture

Because cultural habits inspire most Westerners to sit in a chair when they meditate, floor sitting is usually something folks have to work up to with practice. Over time, your *asana* practice can help you build comfort with sitting on the floor for exercises. As Figure 6-1 shows, your ear, shoulder, and hip are in alignment, as viewed from the side. The following steps walk you through the chair-sitting posture:

1. **Use a sturdy armless chair and sit near the front edge of the seat without leaning against the chair back.**

   Make sure that your feet are flat on the floor. If they don't quite reach, support them with a block, folded blanket, or phone book.

2. **Rest your hands on your knees with your palms down and then close your eyes.**

3. **Rock your spine a few times, alternately slumping forward and arching back to explore its full range of motion.**

   Settle into a comfortable upright position midway between the two extremes.

4. **Lift your chest, without exaggerating the gentle inward curve in your lower back, and balance your head over your torso.**

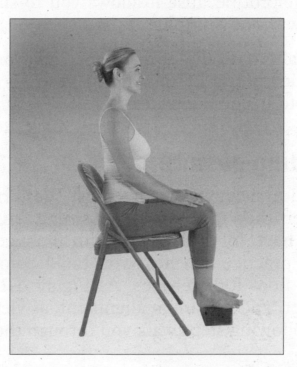

Figure 6-1:
The chair-sitting posture.

The easy posture: Sukhasana

According to Yoga master Patanjali, posture should be "steady" *(sthira)* and "easeful" *(sukha)*. The basic Yoga sitting position is called, appropriately, the easy/easeful posture *(sukhasana),* which Westerners sometimes call the *tailor's seat.* We strongly recommend that beginners start their floor sitting practice with the easy posture, which we illustrate in Figure 6-2.

The easy posture is a steady and comfortable sitting position for meditation and breathing exercises. The posture also helps you become more aware of and actually increase the flexibility in your hips and spine and is therefore a good preparation for more advanced postures.

Here's how it works:

1. **Sit on the floor with your legs straight out in front of you.**

    Place your hands on the floor beside your hips with your palms down and fingers pointing forward; shake your legs up and down a few times to get the kinks out.

2. **Cross your legs at the ankles with the left leg on top, the right leg below.**

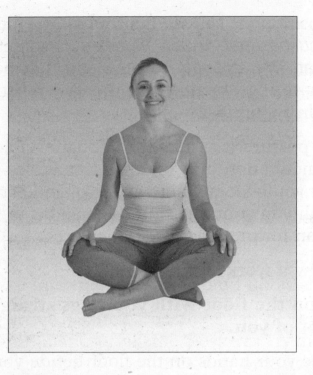

Figure 6-2:
Be sure that you're steady and comfortable in the easy posture.

3. **Press your palms on the floor and slide each foot toward the opposite knee, until your right foot is underneath your left knee and your left foot is underneath your right knee.**

4. **Lengthen the spine by stretching your back in an upward motion and balance your head over your torso.**

Note: In the *classic* (traditionally taught) posture, you drop your chin to your chest and extend your arms and lock your elbows; we suggest, however, that you rest your hands on your knees with your palms down and elbows bent, and keep your head upright, which is more relaxing for beginners.

The thunderbolt posture: Vajrasana

The thunderbolt posture is one of the safer sitting postures for students with back problems. *Vajrasana* increases the flexibility of your ankles, knees, and thighs, improves circulation to the abdomen, and is good for digestion.

Use the following steps to practice this posture:

1. **Kneel on the floor and sit back on your heels.**

   Position each heel under the buttock on the same side and rest your hands on the tops of your knees with your elbows bent and palms down.

2. **Lengthen your spine by stretching your back in an upward motion, balance your head over your torso, and look straight ahead as shown in Figure 6-3.**

Figure 6-3:
A safe sitting posture for lower back problems.

163

Note: In the classic posture, which we don't recommend for beginners, you rest your chin on your upper chest and extend your arms until your elbows are locked and your hands are on your knees.

If you have trouble sitting back on your heels because of tightness in your thigh muscles or pain in your knees, put a cushion or folded blanket between your thighs and calves. Increase the thickness of your lift until you can sit down comfortably. If you feel discomfort in the fronts of your ankles, put a rolled-up towel or blanket underneath them.

The Sanskrit word *vajra* (pronounced *vahj-rah*) means "thunderbolt" or "adamantine." So, this posture is also known as the *adamantine posture.*

The auspicious posture: Svastikasana

Before its perversion in Nazi Germany, the *svastika* served as a solar symbol for good fortune. This is also its meaning in Yoga. The term is made up of the prefix *su* ("good") and *asti* ("is"): "It's good."

The *svastikasana* improves the flexibility of the hips, knees, and ankles and strengthens the back. The following instructions help you get the hang of this posture.

Use the preparation series for advanced sitting postures in Chapter 6 to improve your performance for this posture.

1. **Sit on the floor with your legs straight out in front of you; place your hands on the floor beside your hips with your palms down and fingers pointing forward.**

   Shake your legs up and down a few times to get the kinks out.

2. **Bend your left knee and place the left foot sole against the inside of your right thigh with your left heel close to your groin.**

   If this step is difficult, don't use this pose.

3. **Bend your right knee toward you and take hold of your right foot with both hands.**

4. **Grip the front of your ankle with your right hand and the ball of your big toe with your left; slide the little-toe side of your foot between your left thigh and calf until only your big toe is visible, wiggling the big-toe side of your left foot up between the right thigh and calf if you can.**

5. **Rest your hands on your knees with your arms relaxed and palms down.**

6. **Lengthen your spine by stretching your back in an upward motion, balance your head over your torso, and look straight ahead as illustrated in Figure 6-4.**

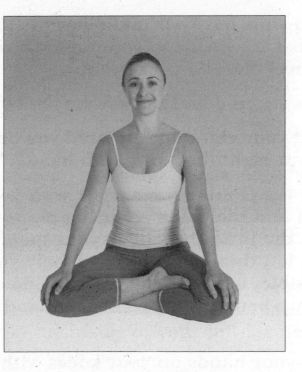

Figure 6-4:
The auspicious posture.

Note: In the classic posture, the chin rests on the chest with the arms straight down and palms open in *jnana mudra* at the knees. The bottom or left foot is pulled up and wedged between the right calf and thigh.

Jnana mudra (pronounced *gyah-nah moo-drah*) or "wisdom seal" is one of a number of hand positions used in Yoga. To do this *mudra,* bring the tip of your index finger to the tip of your thumb to form a circle; extend the three remaining fingers, keeping them close together (as shown in Figure 6-5). This hand gesture makes a good circuit, sealing off the life energy *(prana)* in your body. (Check out Chapter 5 for more on *prana.)*

The perfect posture: Siddhasana

The Sanskrit word *siddha* (pronounced *sidd-hah*) means both "perfect" and "adept." In Yoga, an *adept* isn't just a skillful practitioner but an accomplished master who has attained inner freedom.

Many Yoga masters in bygone eras preferred this posture and used it often in place of the lotus posture. We don't cover either the half lotus or the full lotus position in this book because they're suitable only for more experienced students.

Figure 6-5:
This hand position seals off life energy called *prana.*

The *siddhasana* improves the flexibility of your hips, knees, and ankles, and strengthens the back. The posture is considered the perfect meditation posture for those practicing celibacy. *Siddhasana* is also beneficial for men with various prostate problems.

The preparation series for advanced sitting postures in Chapter 6 can help you with this posture.

Here's how you do it:

1. **Sitting on the floor with your legs straight out**

in front of you, place your hands at your sides (close to your hips) with your palms down and fingers forward.

Shake your legs out in front of you a few times.

2. **Bend your left knee and bring your left heel into your groin near the *perineum* (the area between the anus and the genitals).**

   Stabilize your left ankle with your left hand.

3. **Bend your right knee and slide your right heel towards the front of your left ankle.**

4. **Lift your right foot, position your right ankle just above your left ankle, and bring your right heel into the genital area.**

5. **Tuck the little-toe side of your right foot between your left thigh and calf.**

6. **Place your hands palms down on the same-side knee with arms relaxed.**

7. **Straighten and extend your back and neck, bringing your head up nice and tall; look straight ahead as shown in Figure 6-6.**

   You can use a cushion to raise your hips so that they're level with your knees.

Note: In the classic posture, which we don't recommend for beginners, your chin rests on your chest, your arms are straight down, elbows locked, with your palms open in *jnana mudra* (discussed in the preceding section) at your knees. The big-toe side of your left foot is pulled up and wedged between your right calf and thigh.

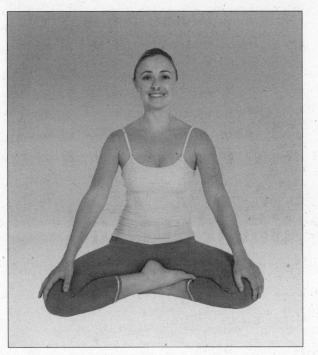

Figure 6-6:
The perfect
posture.

Chapter 7

Standing Tall

Standing upright is a uniquely human trait, and Yoga is a uniquely human practice. In this chapter, we discuss standing from the Yoga perspective, with an emphasis on the difference between just standing and the more quintessential version of *standing*. The simple act of standing upright brings your spine, muscles, tendons, and ligaments into play. Ordinarily, these parts do their assigned tasks quite automatically. But in order to stand efficiently and elegantly, you also need to bring awareness to the act, and that's where Yoga enters the picture.

In this chapter, we give you ten of the more common and favored Yoga standing postures to practice. They can help you discover the art of standing consciously, efficiently, and beautifully.

Identifying That Two-Legged Creature

We are human in large part because hundreds of thousands of years ago our ancestors figured out how to literally stand on their own two feet. Appropriately, the yogic standing postures make up the foundation of *asana* practice.

The way that you stand tells a lot about you. These days, a person who stands tall usually sucks in the belly and sticks out the chest and chin in military fashion. But you can stand tall and straight and be relaxed at the same time.

Body and mind form a unit; they're the outside and the inside of the same person: you. In a way, your body is a map of your mind.

Through regular Yoga practice, you can use the feedback from your body to discipline your mind, and the feedback from your mind (particularly your emotions) to train your body.

Standing Strong

The standing postures are a kind of microcosm of the practice of *asana* as a whole (except for inversions, or upside-down postures, described in Chapter 10); you may

You're grounded!

Calling yogic standing posture an *asana* ("seat") may seem contradictory, but the posture actually helps you become firmly grounded. In Yoga, grounding is as important as reaching up. You can reach the heights of Yoga only when you're as sturdy as a mountain or a sequoia.

hear that you can derive everything you need to know to master your physical practice from the standing postures. The standing postures help you strengthen your legs and ankles, open your hips and groin, and improve your sense of balance. In turn, you develop the ability to "stand your ground" and to "stand at ease," which is an important aspect of the yogic lifestyle.

 The standing postures are very versatile. You can use them in the following ways:

- ✔ As a general warm-up for your practice.

- ✔ In preparation for a specific group of postures (we like to think of the standing forward bends, for example, as a kind of on-ramp to the seated forward bends).

- ✔ For compensation (or to counterbalance another posture, such as a back bend or side bend). For more information, see Chapter 15.

- ✔ For rest.

- ✔ As the main body of your practice.

 You can creatively adapt many postures from other groups to a standing position, which you can then use as a learning (or teaching) tool, or for therapeutic purposes. Take, for example, the well-known cobra posture, a back bend that many beginning students find hard on the lower back (see Chapter 11). By performing this same posture in a standing position near a wall, you can use the changed relationship to gravity, the freedom of not having your hips blocked by the floor, and the pressure of the hands on the wall to free the lower back. Then you can apply this newly won understanding about the back in your practice of the more demanding traditional form of the cobra posture or any other posture that you choose to modify at the wall.

Exercising Your Options

In this section, we introduce you to ten standing postures and describe the step-by-step process for each exercise. We also discuss the benefits and the *classic* (traditionally taught) version of the posture. We don't recommend the

Now, that's a stretch!

A beautiful young woman named Heather came to one of my (Larry's) beginners' Yoga class in Brentwood, California, for her "first ever" Yoga class. It was clear right away that she wasn't very flexible; in fact, she was perhaps the most inflexible young person I'd ever seen. When I led the class in seated forward bends, for example, she literally couldn't touch her knees. In that moment, when she realized how tight she really was, she began to cry. I spoke to her after class and learned that she had been involved in competitive sports since age 5, and that now, at 17, she played on a state champion volleyball team. As athletic as she was, she had done very little stretching over the years . . . and it showed.

I recommended that she lean her buttocks against a wall with her feet about 3 feet away from the wall and just hang down, keeping her knees "soft," as in Forgiving Limbs (covered in Chapter 3). In this modified standing posture, she had an easy angle to bend forward and release her back and hamstrings. She practiced this standing posture every day and within three weeks, she experienced a dramatic change. For the first time, she could sit with her legs extended and reach her toes. With the entire class spontaneously applauding, Heather cried again, but this time out of joy.

classic version for beginners because, in most cases, the postures are more difficult and sometimes risky. Here are a few tips before you get started with the standing postures:

- ✔ Many of these postures start in the mountain posture, so be sure to check out the "Mountain posture: Tadasana" section.

- ✔ When you try the postures on your own, follow the instructions for each exercise carefully, including the breathing. Always move into and out of the posture slowly and pause after the inhalation and exhalation (flip to Chapter 5 for more on breathing). Complete each posture by relaxing and returning to the starting place.

- ✔ When you bend forward from all the standing postures, start with your legs straight (without locking your knees) and then soften your knees when you feel the muscles pulling in the back of your legs.

- ✔ When you come up out of a standing forward bend, choose one of three ways:

  - The easiest and safest way is to roll your body up like a rag doll, stacking your vertebrae one on top of other with your head coming up last.

  - The next level of difficulty is to bring your arms up from the sides like wings as you inhale and raise your back.

  - The third and most challenging way is to start with the inhalation and extend your arms forward and up alongside of the ears. Then continue raising the upper, mid, and lower back until you're straight up and your arms are overhead if possible.

174

Mountain posture: Tadasana

The mountain posture is the foundation for all the standing postures. *Tadasana* aligns the body, improves posture and balance, and facilitates breathing. Although this exercise is commonly called the mountain posture, the name for this position is actually "palm posture," from the Sanskrit word *tada* (pronounced *tah-dah*). Some authorities also refer to this exercise as the tree posture. Here's how it works:

1. **Stand tall but relaxed with your feet at hip width (down from the sits bones, not the outer curves) and hang your arms at your sides, palms turned toward your legs.**

   The *sits bones,* also know as the *ischial tuberosity,* are the bony parts you feel underneath you when you sit up straight on a firm surface.

2. **Visualize a vertical line connecting the opening in your ear, your shoulder joint, and the sides of your hip, knee, and ankle.**

   Look straight ahead, with your eyes open or closed as shown in Figure 7-1.

3. **Remain in this posture for 6 to 8 breaths.**

Note: In the classic version of this posture, the feet are together, and the chin rests on the chest.

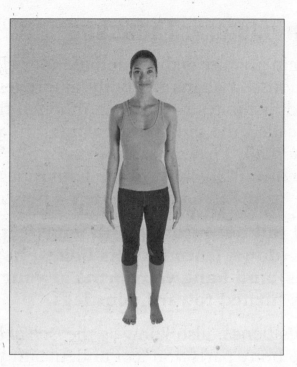

Figure 7-1:
Start your standing postures with the mountain posture.

Standing forward bend: Uttanasana

The Sanskrit word *uttana* (pronounced *oo-tah-nah*) means "extended," and this posture certainly fits that bill. The standing forward bend (see Figure 7-2) stretches the entire back of the body and decompresses the neck (makes space between the vertebrae). In the upright posture, the cervical spine and the neck muscles work hard to balance the head. Because most people generally don't pay enough attention to this part of their anatomy, they tend to accumulate a lot of tension in their necks, which can lead to headaches. This posture frees the cervical spine and allows the neck muscles to relax. It also improves overall circulation and has a calming effect on the body and mind. The following steps walk you through the process.

176

Be very careful of all forward bends if you're having a disc problem. If you're unsure, check with your doctor or health professional.

1. **Start in mountain posture and as you inhale, raise your arms forward and then up overhead (see Figure 7-2a).**

2. **As you exhale, bend forward from your hips.**

   When you feel a pull in the back of your legs, soften your knees (as in the Forgiving Limbs discussion in Chapter 3) and hang your arms.

3. **If your head isn't close to your knees, bend your knees more.**

   If you have the flexibility, straighten your knees but keep them soft. Relax your head and neck downward as Figure 7-2b illustrates.

4. **As you inhale, roll up slowly, stacking the bones of your spine one at a time from bottom to top and then raise your arms overhead.**

   Rolling is the safest way to come up. If you don't have back problems, after a few weeks you may want to try the two more advanced techniques we discuss earlier in the section.

5. **Repeat Steps 1 through 4 three times and then stay in the folded position (Step 3) for 6 to 8 breaths.**

Note: In the classic posture, the feet are together and the legs are straight. The forehead presses against the shins, and the palms are on the floor.

Figure 7-2:
The standing forward bend.

a b

Half standing forward bend: Ardha uttanasana

The Sanskrit word *ardha* (pronounced *ahrd-ha*) means "half." The half standing forward bend strengthens your legs, back, shoulders, and arms and improves stamina. Here's how you do it:

1. **Start in the mountain posture and as you inhale, raise your arms forward and then up overhead as in the standing forward bend (see the preceding section).**

2. **As you exhale, bend forward from your hips.**

   Soften your knees and hang your arms.

3. **Bend your knees, and as you inhale, raise your torso and arms up from the front so that**

they're parallel to the floor as shown in Figure 7-3.

If you have any back problems, keep your arms back by your sides, and then over a period of time gradually stretch them out to the sides like a *T* and eventually in front of you so they're parallel to the floor.

4. **Bring your head to a neutral position so that your ears are between your arms.**

Look down and a little forward. To make the posture easier, move your arms back toward your hips — the further back, the easier.

5. **Repeat Steps 1 through 4 three times and then stay in Step 4 for 6 to 8 breaths.**

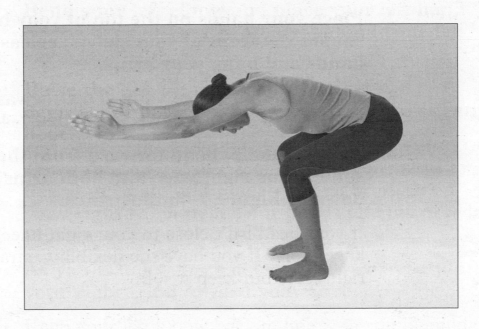

Figure 7-3:
The half standing forward bend is great for stamina.

Note: In the classical version of this posture, the feet are together and the legs and arms are straight.

Asymmetrical forward bend: Parshva uttanasana

The asymmetrical forward bend stretches each side of the back and hamstrings separately. The Sanskrit word *parshva* (pronounced *pahr-shvah*) means "side" or "flank," and this posture indeed opens the hips, tones the abdomen, decompresses the neck, improves balance, and increases circulation to the upper torso and head.

1. **Stand in the mountain posture and as you exhale, step forward about 3 to 3 1/2 feet (or the length of one leg) with your right foot.**

    Your left foot turns out naturally, but if you need more stability turn it out more (so that the toes point to the left.)

2. **Place your hands on the top of your hips and square the front of your pelvis; release your hands and hang your arms.**

3. **As you inhale, raise your arms forward and then overhead as shown in Figure 7-4a.**

4. **As you exhale, bend forward from the hips, soften your right knee and both arms, and hang down as Figure 7-4b illustrates.**

    If your head isn't close to your right knee, bend your knee more. If you have the flexibility, straighten your right knee but keep it soft.

Figure 7-4:
This exercise stretches each side of the back and hamstrings separately.

5. **As you inhale, roll up slowly, stacking the bones of your spine one at a time from the bottom up, and then raise your arms overhead.**

   Relax your head and neck downward. Rolling up is the safest way to come up but if you don't have back problems, you may want to try the more advanced techniques we cover earlier in the section after a few weeks.

6. **Repeat Steps 3 and 4 three times and then stay in Step 4 for 6 to 8 breaths.**

   Repeat the same sequence on the left side.

Note: In the classic version of this posture, both legs are straight and the forehead presses against the forward leg.

To make the posture more challenging, square your hips forward and rotate your back foot inward.

Triangle posture: Utthita trikonasana

The Sanskrit word *utthita* (pronounced *oot-hee-tah*) means "raised" and *trikona* (pronounced *tree-ko-nah*) means "triangle." The latter term is often mispronounced as *try-ko-nah*. The triangle posture stretches the sides of your spine, the backs of your legs, and your hips. It also stretches the muscles between your ribs (the *intercostals*), which opens the chest and improves breathing capacity. Just follow these steps:

1. **Stand in the mountain posture, exhale, and step out to the right about 3 to 3 1/2 feet (or the length of one leg) with your right foot.**

2. **Turn your right foot out 90 degrees and your left foot 45 degrees.**

    An imaginary line drawn from the right heel (toward the left foot) should bisect the arch of the left foot.

3. **Face forward and, as you inhale, raise your arms out to the sides parallel to the line of the shoulders (and the floor) so that they form a *T* with the torso (see Figure 7-5a).**

4. **As you exhale, reach your right hand down to your right shin as close to the ankle as is comfortable for you and then reach and lift your left arm up.**

    Bend your right knee slightly as shown in Figure 7-5b if the back of your leg feels tight. As much as you can, bring the sides of your torso parallel to the floor.

5. **Soften your left arm and look up at your left hand.**

    If your neck hurts, look down or halfway down at the floor.

6. Repeat Steps 3 through 5 three times and then stay in Step 5 for 6 to 8 breaths.

Repeat the same sequence on the left side.

Note: In the classic version of this posture, the feet are parallel, the arms and legs are straight, and the trunk is parallel to the floor. The right hand is on the floor outside the right foot.

Figure 7-5:
The side-bending triangle opens the chest so you can breathe deeply.

Reverse triangle posture: Parivritta trikonasana

The Sanskrit word *parivritta* (pronounced *pah-ree-vree-tah*) means "revolved," which makes perfect sense with this posture. The action of twists, including the reverse triangle, on the discs between the spinal vertebrae (intervertebral discs) is often compared to squeezing and then releasing a wet sponge: First you squeeze the dirty water out and then you sponge up the clean water. The twisting-untwisting action increases circulation of fresh blood to these discs and keeps them supple as you grow older. The reverse triangle

183

also stretches the backs of your legs, opens your hips, and strengthens your neck, shoulders, and arms. Here's how it works:

1. **Standing in the mountain posture, exhale and step the right foot out to the right about 3 to 3 1/2 feet (or the length of one leg).**

2. **As you inhale, raise your arms out to the sides parallel to the line of the shoulders (and the floor) so that they form a *T* with the torso as Figure 7-6a illustrates.**

3. **As you exhale, bend forward from the hips and then place the right hand on the floor near the inside of the left foot.**

4. **Raise your left arm toward the ceiling and look up at your left hand.**

   Soften your knees and your arms. Bend your left knee or move your right hand away from your left foot (and more directly under your torso) as in Figure 7-6b if necessary. If you feel neck strain, turn your head toward the floor.

5. **Repeat Steps 2 through 4 three times and then stay in Step 4 for 6 to 8 breaths.**

   Repeat the same sequence on the left side.

Figure 7-6:
The reverse triangle posture.

Note: In the classic version of this posture, the feet are parallel and the legs and arms are straight. The torso is parallel to the floor and the bottom hand rests lightly outside the opposite side foot.

Warrior I: Vira bhadrasana I

The Sanskrit word *vira* (pronounced *vee-rah*) is often translated as "hero" and *bhadra* (pronounced *bhud-rah*) means "auspicious." This posture, also known as just *warrior,* strengthens your legs, back, shoulders, and arms; opens your hips, groin, and chest; increases strength and stamina; and improves balance. As its name suggests, this posture instills a feeling of fearlessness and inner strength. The following steps get you going:

1. **Stand in the mountain posture and as you exhale, step forward approximately 3 to 3 1/2 feet (or the length of one leg) with your right foot (see Figure 7-7a).**

    Your left foot turns out naturally, but if you need more stability, turn it out more (so that your toes point to the left).

2. **Place your hands on the top of your hips and square the front of your pelvis; release your hands and hang your arms.**

3. **As you inhale, raise your arms forward and overhead and bend your right knee to a right angle (so that the knee is directly over the ankle and the thigh is parallel to the floor) as shown in Figure 7-7b.**

   If your lower back is uncomfortable, lean the torso slightly over the forward leg until you feel a release of tension in your back.

4. **As you exhale, return to the starting place in Figure 7-7a; soften your arms and face your palms toward each other, looking straight ahead.**

5. **Repeat Steps 3 and 4 three times and then stay in Step 3 for 6 to 8 breaths.**

6. **Repeat Steps 1 through 5 on the left side.**

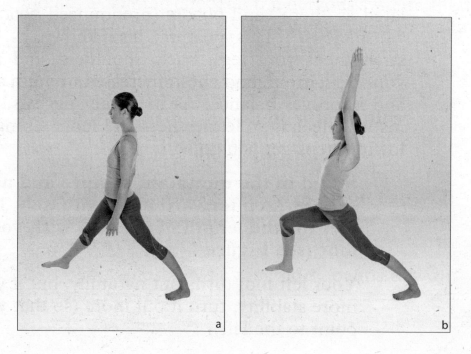

Figure 7-7:
The warrior is a position of power and strength.

Warrior II: Vira bhadrasana II

Like the warrior I posture we cover in the preceding section, warrior II also strengthens your legs, back, shoulders, and arms. It focuses more on your hips and groin and increases strength and stamina; it also improves balance. Use the following steps as your guide.

1. **Stand in the mountain posture; exhale, and step out to the right about 3 to 3 1/2 feet (or the length of one leg) with your right foot.**

2. **Turn your right foot out 90 degrees and your left foot 45 degrees.**

   An imaginary line drawn from your right heel toward your left foot should bisect the arch of your left foot.

3. **Face forward and, as you inhale, raise your arms out to the sides parallel to the line of the shoulders (and the floor) so that they form a *T* with the torso (see Figure 7-8a).**

4. **As you exhale, turn your right foot out 90 degrees and bend your right knee over your right ankle so that your shin is perpendicular to the floor as shown in see Figure 7-8b.**

   If possible, bring the right thigh parallel to the floor.

5. **Repeat Steps 3 and 4 three times, keeping your arms in a *T*, and then turn your head to the right, looking out over your right arm, and stay for 6 to 8 breaths.**

6. **Repeat Steps 1 through 5 on the left side.**

Be careful not to force your hips open — it may cause problems with your knees (and you don't want that!).

Figure 7-8:
Warrior II.

Standing spread-legged forward bend: Prasarita pada uttanasana

The Sanskrit word *prasarita* (pronounced *prah-sah-ree-tah*) means "outstretched" and *pada,* (pronounced *pah-dah*) means "foot." This posture, also called the wide-legged standing forward bend, stretches your hamstrings and your *adductors* (on insides of the thighs) and opens your hips. The hanging forward bend increases circulation to your upper torso and lengthens your spine. Figure 7-9 shows you this posture; here's how you do it:

1. **Stand in the mountain posture, exhale, and step your right foot out to the right about 3 to 3 1/2 feet (or the length of one leg).**

2. **As you inhale, raise your arms out to the sides parallel to the line of your shoulders (and the floor) so they form a *T* with your torso.**

3. **As you exhale, bend forward from the hips and soften your knees.**

4. **Hold your bent elbows with the opposite-side**

hands and hang your torso and arms.

5. **Stay in Step 4 for 6 to 8 breaths.**

Figure 7-9:
A great way to release pressure in your lower back.

Note: In the classic version of this posture, the legs are straight, the head is on the floor (and the chin presses the chest), and the arms reach back between the legs, palms on the floor.

Half chair posture: Ardha utkatasana

The Sanskrit word *ardha* (pronounced *ahrd-ha*) means "half," and *utkata,* (pronounced *oot-kah-tah*) translates as "extraordinary." The half chair posture strengthens the back, legs, shoulders, and arms and builds overall stamina. If you find this posture difficult or have problem knees, you may want to skip this position for now and return to it after your leg muscles become a little stronger. Don't overdo this exercise (either by holding the position too long or by

189

repeating it more than we recommend), or you'll have sore muscles the next day. But there's no harm in experiencing some muscle soreness either, especially if you haven't exercised in a long time. Check out Figure 7-10 and the following steps for guidance.

1. **Start in the mountain posture and as you inhale, raise your arms forward and up overhead with palms facing each other.**

2. **As you exhale, bend your knees and squat halfway to the floor.**

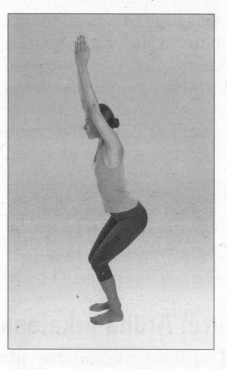

Figure 7-10: The half chair is a great posture for overall stamina.

3. **Soften your arms but keep them overhead.**

Look straight ahead.

4. **Repeat Steps 1 through 3 three times and then stay in Step 3 for 6 to 8 breaths.**

Note: In the classic version of this posture, the feet are together and the arms are straight, with the fingers inter-locked and the palms turned upward. The chin rests on the chest.

Downward-facing dog: Adhomukha shvanasana

The Sanskrit word *adhomukha* (pronounced *ahd-ho-mook-hah*) means "downward facing," and *shvan* (pronounced *shvahn*) means "dog." Yoga masters were great observers of the world around them. They particularly noticed the behavior of animals, which is why the dog's leisurely stretching inspired them to create a similar posture for humans. The practice of downward-facing dog stretches the entire back of your body, and strengthens your wrists, arms, and shoulders. This posture is a good alternative for beginning students who aren't yet ready for inversions like the handstand and headstand. Because the head is lower than the heart, this *asana* circulates fresh blood to the brain and acts as a quick pick-me-up when you're fatigued.

1. **Start on your hands and knees; straighten your arms, but don't lock your elbows (see Figure 7-11a).**

   Be sure that the heels of your hands are directly under your shoulders, with your palms on the floor with the fingers spread and your knees directly under your hips. Emphasize pressing down with the thumbs and index fingers or the inner web of your hand.

2. **As you exhale, lift and straighten (but don't lock) your knees.**

   As your hips lift, bring your head to a neutral

191

position so that your ears are between your arms.

3. **Press your heels toward the floor and your head toward your feet as in Figure 7-11b.**

Don't complete this step if doing so strains your neck.

4. **Repeat Steps 1 through 3 three times and then stay in Step 3 for 6 to 8 breaths.**

Note: In the classic posture, the feet are together and flat on the floor, the legs and arms are straight, and the top of the head is on the floor with the chin pressed to the chest.

Be careful not to hold this posture too long if you have problems with your neck, shoulders, wrists, or elbows.

Figure 7-11: *Challenge yourself in downward-facing dog, but don't strain.*

Chapter 8

Steady as a Tree:
Mastering Balance

- -

In This Chapter

▶ Understanding the psychology of balance
▶ Practicing balancing exercises

- -

Balance (called *samata [sah-mah-tah]* or *samatva [sah-mah-tvah]* in Sanskrit) is fundamental to Yoga. A balanced approach to life includes being even-tempered and seeing the great unity behind all diversity. Balance translates to being nonjudgmental and treating others with equal fairness, kindness, and compassion.

One way to begin to gain this balance is to practice balancing postures. Remember, according to Yoga, body and mind form a working unit. Imbalances in the body are reflected in the mind, and vice versa. This chapter emphasizes the importance of balance in Yoga and offers six postures that provide you with a *samata* sampling.

193

Getting to the Roots of the Posture

When you look at a tree, you see only what is above ground — the vertical trunk with its crown of branches and foliage and maybe a few chirping birds. Trees appear to just perch atop the soil, and you wonder how in the world such a top-heavy thing can stay upright.

Well, everyone knows that the secret of the tree's equilibrium is its underground network of roots that anchor the visible part of the plant solidly into the earth. In the balancing postures, you too can discover how to grow your "roots" into the earth and stand up as steady as a tree.

For us, the balancing postures can be the most fun and the most dramatic of all the postures. Although they're relatively simple, the postures can produce profound effects. As you may expect, they work to improve your overall sense of physical balance, coordination, and grounding. With awareness in these three areas, you can move more easily and effectively, whether you're going about your daily business or are engaged in activities calling for great coordination, such as sports or dance. The yogic balancing postures also have therapeutic applications, such as with back problems or retraining whole muscle groups.

 When you improve your physical balance naturally, you can expect to enjoy improved mental balance. The balancing postures are exceptional seeds for concentration, and when they're mastered, they create confidence and a sense of accomplishment.

Balancing Postures for Graceful Strength

Contemporary life is highly demanding and stressful; if you're not properly grounded, you face a constant risk of being pushed out of balance. *Grounding* means being centered and firm without being inflexible, knowing who you are and what you want, and feeling that you're empowered to achieve your life goals. A good way to begin your grounding work is by improving your physical sense of balance, which helps you synchronize the movement of your arms and legs, giving you poise. When you can stand and move in a more balanced manner, your mind is automatically affected. You *feel* more balanced.

A sense of balance is connected with the inner ears. Your ears tell you where you are in space. The ears are also connected with *social space;* if you aren't well-balanced, you may feel — or actually *be* — a bit awkward in your social relationships. Balancing and grounding work can remedy this discomfort. Only when you can stand still — in balance — can you also move harmoniously in the world.

The following postures appear in order of easier to more advanced exercises. If you try the postures individually rather than as part of a sequence, we recommend that you hold each posture for 6 to 8 breaths. Breathe freely through the nose and pause briefly after inhalation and exhalation.

Warrior at the wall: Vira bhadrasana III variation

The Sanskrit word *vira* (pronounced *vee-rah*) means "hero." *Bhadra* (pronounced *bhud-rah*) means "auspicious." This posture improves your overall balance and stability. It strengthens the legs, arms, and shoulders and stretches the thighs — both front and back — and the hips. As with the other one-legged balancing poses, this posture enhances focus and concentration. Check out the following steps:

1. **Stand in the mountain posture (see Chapter 7),**

facing a blank wall about three feet away.

2. **As you exhale, bend forward from the hips and extend your arms forward until your fingertips are touching the wall.**

   Adjust yourself so that your legs are perpendicular and your torso and arms are parallel with the floor.

3. **As you inhale, raise your left leg back and up until it's parallel to the floor (see Figure 8-1).**

4. **Stay in Step 3 for 6 to 8 breaths; repeat with the right leg.**

Figure 8-1:
A safe balancing posture for beginners.

Balancing cat

Balancing cat strengthens the muscles along the spine (the *paraspinals*), as well as the arms, and the shoulders, and it opens the hips. The posture enhances focus and concentration and also builds confidence.

1. **Beginning on your hands and knees, position your hands directly under your shoulders with your palms down, your fingers spread on the floor, and your knees directly under your hips.**

   Straighten your arms, but don't lock your elbows.

2. **As you exhale, slide your left hand forward and your right leg back, keeping your hand and your toes on the floor.**

3. **As you inhale, raise your left arm and right leg to a comfortable height as Figure 8-2 illustrates.**

4. **Stay in Step 3 for 6 to 8 breaths and then repeat Steps 1 through 3 with opposite pairs (right arm and left leg).**

This posture is a variation of *cakravakasana* (pronounced *chuk-rah-vahk-ah-sah-nah*). The *cakravaka* is a particular kind of goose, which in India's traditional poetry is often used to convey "love bird." Apparently, when these birds have paired up and then are separated, their heartache causes them to call to each other.

Figure 8-2:
Extend your arm and leg fully on the ground before you lift them up.

197

The tree posture: Vrikshasana

The Sanskrit word *vriksha* (pronounced *vrik-shah*) means "tree." The tree posture improves overall balance, stability, and poise. It strengthens your legs, arms, and shoulders, and opens your hips and groin. Like the other one-legged balancing poses, it also enhances focus and concentration and produces a calming effect on your body and mind. Here's how it works:

1. **Stand in the mountain posture (covered in Chapter 7).**

2. **As you exhale, bend your right knee and place the sole of your right foot, toes pointing down, on the inside of your left leg between your knee and your groin.**

3. **As you inhale, bring your arms over your head and join your palms together.**

4. **Soften your arms and focus on a spot 6 to 8 feet in front of you on the floor as shown in Figure 8-3.**

5. **Stay in Step 4 for 6 to 8 breaths and then repeat with the opposite leg.**

Note: In the *classic* (traditionally taught) version of this posture, the arms are straight and the chin rests on the chest.

Figure 8-3:
Focus on a spot 6 to 8 feet in front of you; concentrate and breathe slowly.

The karate kid

The karate kid improves overall balance and stability. It strengthens the legs, arms, and shoulders and opens the hips. As with the other one-legged balancing postures, the karate kid enhances focus and concentration. Just follow these steps:

1. **Stand in the mountain posture, which we describe in Chapter 7.**

2. **As you inhale, raise your arms out to the sides parallel to the line of your shoulders (and the floor) so that they form a *T* with your torso.**

3. **To steady yourself, focus on a spot on the floor 10 to 12 feet in front of you.**

4. **As you exhale, bend your left knee, raising it toward your chest.**

199

Keep your right leg straight (see Figure 8-4).

5. **Stay in Step 4 for 6 to 8 breaths; repeat with the right knee.**

Figure 8-4:
The karate kid.

The Sanskrit name for this pose would be "utthita hasta padangusthasana variation." I (Larry) called it the karate kid based on inspiration from the film *The Karate Kid, Part II.*

Standing heel-to-buttock

The standing heel-to-buttock posture improves your overall balance and stability. This posture strengthens your legs, arms, and shoulders and stretches your thighs. As with the other one-legged balancing poses, this posture enhances focus and concentration. Here's how it works

1. **Stand in the mountain posture (see Chapter 7).**

2. **As you inhale, raise your left arm forward and overhead.**

3. **To steady yourself, focus on a spot on the floor 10 to 12 feet in front of you.**

4. **As you exhale, bend your right knee and bring your right heel toward your right buttock, keeping your left leg straight.**

   Grasp your right ankle with the right hand as Figure 8-5 illustrates.

5. **Stay in Step 4 for 6 to 8 breaths; repeat Steps 1 through 5 with your left foot.**

Figure 8-5:
This pose can improve your balance for the more advanced postures.

Scorpion

The scorpion posture improves overall balance and stability. This posture, which is a variation of *cakravakasana*, strengthens your shoulders, improves the flexibility of your hips, legs, and shoulders, and enhances focus and concentration. The following steps walk you through the process:

1. **While on your hands and knees, position your hands directly under your shoulders with your palms down, fingers spread on the floor, and your knees directly under your hips.**

   Straighten your arms, but don't lock your elbows.

2. **Place your right forearm on the floor with your right hand just behind your left wrist.**

   Reach behind you with your left hand, twisting the torso slightly to the left, and grab your right ankle.

3. **As you inhale, lift your right knee off the floor, raise your chest until it's parallel to the floor, and look up.**

   Find a comfortable height for your chest and raised leg. Steady yourself by pressing your right forearm and thumb on the floor (see Figure 8-6).

4. **Stay in Step 3 for 6 to 8 breaths and then repeat Steps 1 through 4 on the opposite side (left forearm and left foot).**

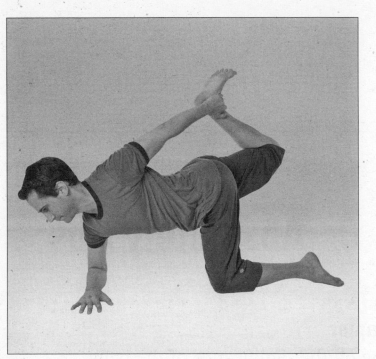

Figure 8-6:
Steady yourself by pressing your right forearm and thumb into the floor.

Chapter 9

Absolutely Abs

Many Eastern systems of spiritual exercise and healing consider the lower abdomen to be the vital center of your whole being — body, mind, and spirit. Westerners, on the other hand, think much differently about their bellies, tending to see them as mere food bags or as waste processing stations.

Many people have a love-hate relationship with their bellies. Although people may be obsessed with having the "perfect" midriff, they tend to neglect or even abuse this area of their bodies. On the inside, they stuff the belly with way too much junk food. On the outside, they let it grow slack. But, as the Yoga masters warn, when this area is polluted by impurities, it becomes a seat of sickness.

Apart from diseases, weak bellies (and belly muscles) contribute significantly to lower back problems. Studies indicate that 80 percent of the American population has had, is having, or will have back problems, and that back-related problems are the second-leading cause of missed workdays, trailing only respiratory problems or the common cold.

In this chapter, we walk you through some Yoga exercises that focus on the abdomen so that you can keep this vital area of your body strong and healthy.

Taking Care of the Abdomen: Your Business Center

The abdomen is an amazing enterprise, with its complex food-processing plant (the stomach), several subsidiary operations (liver, spleen, kidneys, and so on), and a 25-foot-long sewer system (the intestines). Poor diets and eating habits lead to annoying and sometimes deadly serious digestive and elimination problems, including constipation, diarrhea, irritable bowel syndrome, and colon cancer. Regular Yoga practice can help you take care of your abdominal organs so they can function well and take care of you without the aid of antacids, digestive enzyme supplements, or laxatives.

In the following section, we describe exercises that work with three sets of abdominal muscles:

✔ The *rectus abdominis,* which is strung vertically along the front of the belly from the bottom of the sternum to the pubis

✔ The internal and external *obliques,* which, as their name suggests, take an "oblique" course along the side of the belly from the lower ribs to the top rim of the pelvis

✔ The *transversalis abdominis,* which lies behind the internal obliques

You may hear these three abdominals called the "stomach muscles," which is really a misnomer. The actual stomach muscles line the baglike stomach and are active only during digestion. Of course, the yogic exercises also positively affect the abdominal organs (stomach, spleen, liver, and intestines). If you take care of your abdominal muscles and the organs they protect — through exercise and proper diet — you have accomplished 90 percent of the work to stay healthy.

Navel secrets, declassified

After a doctor severs a child's umbilical cord, thus creating his navel, no one pays much attention to this birth socket. Yet the navel is a very important feature of your anatomy. According to Yoga, a special psychoenergetic center is located at the navel. This center is known as the *manipura-cakra* (pronounced *mah-nee-poo-rah-chuk-rah*), which means literally "center of the jeweled city." The center corresponds to (but isn't identical with) the *solar plexus,* which is a large network of nerves that has been called the body's second brain. The *manipura-cakra* controls the abdominal organs and regulates the flow of energy through the entire body. The navel center is associated with emotions and the will. You can have "too much navel" (be pushy) or "not enough navel" (be a pushover).

Exercising Those Abs

Our yogic postures for the abdominal muscles incorporate a team approach that values slow, conscious movement, proper breathing mechanics, and the use of sound. The emphasis here is on the *quality* of the movement rather than sheer quantity. A few movements done with diligent attention are much safer and more effective than dozens and even hundreds of mindless repetitions. Conscious breathing, especially the gentle tightening of the front belly on each exhalation, can encourage and then sustain the strength and tone of the abdominals. The use of sound, which we discuss later in this chapter, further enhances this kind of breathing.

Exploring push-downs

Push-downs strengthen the abdomen, especially the lower abdomen. In addition to a floor exercise, you can do push-downs in a seated position by pushing your lower back against the back of your chair. You can perform this exercise sitting in a car, on a plane, or at the office.

1. **Lie on your back with your knees bent and your feet on the floor at hip width.**

   Rest your arms near your sides, palms down.

2. **As you exhale, push your lower back down to the floor for 3 to 5 seconds (see Figure 9-1).**

3. **As you inhale, release your back.**

4. **Repeat Steps 2 and 3 six to eight times.**

Figure 9-1:
Push your lower back down as you exhale.

Trying yogi sit-ups

Yogi sit-ups strengthen the abdomen, especially the upper abdomen, the *adductors* (insides of your legs), the neck, and the shoulders.

1. **Lie on your back with your knees bent and your feet on the floor at hip width.**

2. **Turn your toes in "pigeon-toed" and bring your inner knees together.**

3. **Spread your palms on the back of your head with your fingers interlocked and keep your elbows wide.**

4. **As you exhale, press your knees firmly, tilt the front of your pelvis toward your navel, and with your hips on the ground, slowly sit up halfway.**

   Keep your elbows out to the sides in line with the tops of your shoulders. Look toward the ceiling. Don't pull your head up with your arms; rather, support your head with your hands and come up by contracting the abdominal muscles as shown in Figure 9-2.

5. As you inhale, slowly roll back down.

6. Repeat Steps 4 and 5 six to eight times.

Figure 9-2:
Let your eyes follow the ceiling as you sit up.

The sound of Yoga

A very busy, well-known movie producer from Malibu was referred to me (Larry) by his physician. He suffered from a chronic neck and stress condition, and also had what his girlfriend referred to as a "little jelly belly." Regular sit-ups to tighten his abs just aggravated his neck problem. I gave him a 12-minute, twice-a-day Yoga routine that included the yogi sit-back and the use of sound (both discussed in this chapter). The exercises worked like a charm. His neck problem went away, his belly firmed up nicely. He liked using sound so much that many members of his movie crew joined him in the afternoon for "a little sound."

Strengthening with yogi sit-backs

Yogi sit-backs strengthen both the lower and upper abdomen. This posture is a variation of *navasana*. The Sanskrit word *nava*, pronounced *nah-vah*, means "boat."

1. **Sit on the floor with your knees bent and your feet on the floor at hip width.**

2. **Place your hands on the floor, palms down, near your hips.**

3. **Bring your chin down and round your back in a C curve like in Figure 9-3a.**

4. **As you inhale, roll slowly onto the back of your pelvis, dragging your hands along on the floor as shown in Figure 9-3b.**

   Keep the rest of your back off the floor to maintain the contraction of the abdominals, but don't strain to hold this position; if you have any negative symptoms, don't use this posture.

5. **As you exhale, roll up again, sliding your hands forward.**

6. **Repeat Steps 4 and 5 six to eight times.**

Figure 9-3:
Bring your chin down and keep your back rounded in a C curve.

Sit-backs are easier on the neck than most sit-ups. However, if you have lower back problems, be cautious with sit-backs. If you notice any pain in your back, just stop. Work with the other exercises in this chapter instead.

Creating variety with extended leg slide-ups

A variation of *navasana*, the extended leg slide-ups strengthen both the upper and lower abdomen as well as the neck.

If this pose bothers your neck, support your head by putting both hands behind it. If the problem persists, stop.

1. **Lie on your back with your knees bent and your feet flat on the floor at hip width.**

2. **Bend your left elbow and place your left hand on the back of your head just behind your left ear.**

3. **Raise the left leg as close to vertical (90 degrees) as possible, but keep your knee slightly bent.**

4. **Draw the top of your foot toward your shin to flex your ankle and place your right palm on your right thigh near your pelvis as Figure 9-4a illustrates.**

5. **As you exhale, sit up slowly halfway and slide your right hand toward your knee.**

   Keep your left elbow back in line with your shoulder and look at the ceiling. Don't throw your head forward (see Figure 9-4b for the proper positioning).

6. **Repeat Steps 1 through 5 six to eight times and**

then repeat Steps 1 through 6 on the other side.

Figure 9-4:
Work the abs and the hamstrings.

Arching with the suck 'em up posture

The suck 'em up posture strengthens and tones the abdominal muscles and the internal organs. The posture is especially beneficial for relieving constipation.

1. **Start on your hands and knees with your hands just below your shoulders and your knees at hip width.**

2. **Inhale deeply through your nose.**

3. **Exhale through your mouth and hump your back like a camel as you bring your chin down.**

   When you have fully exhaled, don't immediately inhale; hold your breath where it is and then suck your belly up towards your spine (see Figure 9-5).

   Wait two to three seconds with the belly up and breath restrained, providing you don't end up gasping for air.

4. **As you inhale, return to the starting position and then pause for a breath or two.**

212

5. **Repeat Steps 2 through 4 four to six times, pausing for a breath or two between each repetition.**

Do this exercise only on an empty stomach, and avoid it if you're having stomach pain or cramps of any kind because it may intensify the symptoms. Avoid this exercise during menstruation.

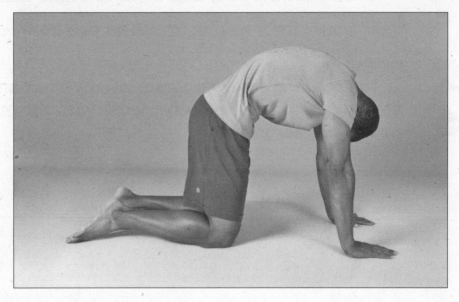

Figure 9-5:
Make sure that you exhale fully before you suck your belly up.

Exhaling "soundly"

The use of sound exercise strengthens and tones the abdomen and its internal organs in addition to strengthening the muscles of the diaphragm.

1. **Sit in a chair or on the floor with your spine comfortably upright.**

   If you find yourself slumping, sit on a folded blanket or check out the Yoga props in Chapter 19.

2. **Place the palm of your right hand on your**

navel so that you can feel your belly contracting as you exhale.

3. **Take a deep inhalation through your nose and, as you exhale, make the sound** *ah, ma,* **or** *sa.*

   Continue sounding this consonant for as long as you can do so comfortably.

4. **Repeat Steps 2 and 3 six to eight times.**

   Pause for a resting breath or two between each sound.

If you're on a detox program of any kind and the use of sound gives you a headache, work with the other exercises in this chapter instead.

Chapter 10

Looking at the World Upside Down

- -

In This Chapter
▶ Making heads or tails of the yogic principle of reversal
▶ Working with leg inversions
▶ Gravitating toward shoulder stands

- -

Thousands of years ago, the Yoga masters made an amazing discovery: By tricking the force of gravity with the help of inversion exercises, you can reverse the effects of aging, improve your health, and add years to your life.

To picture how inversions work, take a look at a jug of unfiltered apple juice sitting on the grocery store shelf. Gravity has pulled the solids in the juice to the bottom of the jug, diluting the liquid near the top. If you turn the bottle upside down, gravity pulls the bottom sediment toward the top of the inverted jug, remixing the juice with the pulp of the apples.

In a similar way, when you turn yourself upside down, the sediments — mostly blood and *lymph* (a clear yellowish fluid similar to blood plasma) — that have collected in your lower limbs during a long day of uprightness sink toward your head and revitalize your entire body and mind, helping you face your fears and reversing the tide of stagnation and mental negativity.

The idea that you must practice the headstand to be a "real yogi" just isn't true. We recommend that you avoid the headstand unless an experienced teacher supervises your efforts. The neck is designed to support the 8 pounds of the head, not the 100 or more pounds of the body. Approach the headstand cautiously and only after proper preparation.

Fortunately, you can practice a variety of inversions other than the headstand. In this chapter, we describe inverted exercises that impart the benefits without the risk. Use yogic breathing (see Chapter 5) to boost their beneficial effect, and grab a prop as necessary to facilitate the postures and ensure easy breathing (see Chapter 19).

Getting a Leg Up on Leg Inversions

Effective inversions can actually be quite simple. In the section below, we describe four postures that don't require you to literally turn yourself upside down in order to enjoy the numerous benefits of an inversion.

 Avoid all inverted postures if you have an acute headache or if you experience sudden pain while performing the exercise.

Legs up on a chair

The legs up on a chair posture improves circulation to your legs, hips, and lower back and has a calming effect on your nervous system. It also helps alleviate symptoms of PMS in women and prostatitis in men.

To enjoy these benefits, do the following:

1. **Sit on the floor in a simple cross-legged position facing a sturdy chair and then lean back onto your forearms.**

2. **Slide your buttocks along the floor toward the chair until they're just under the front edge of the chair seat.**

3. **While exhaling, lift your feet off the floor and place your heels and calves on the chair seat.**

   Make sure that the front edge of the seat is close to the backs of your knees.

4. **Lie back on the floor with your arms near your sides, palms down or up as shown in Figure 10-1.**

5. **Stay in Step 4 for 2 to 10 minutes.**

This posture is a variation of the *classic* (traditionally taught) posture of *urdhva prasarita padasana* (pronounced *oord-hvah prah-sah-ree-tah pahd-ah-sah-nah*) which means "upward extended foot posture."

Figure 10-1:
The legs up on a chair posture.

Legs up on the wall

Legs up on the wall, which is a variation of *urdhva prasarita padasana,* improves circulation to the legs, hips, and lower back and has a calming effect on the nervous system. It also helps alleviate symptoms of PMS in women and prostatitis in men.

Try it for yourself by following these steps:

1. **Sit sideways with your right side as close to the wall as possible, with both legs extended forward as Figure 10-2a illustrates.**

2. **As you exhale, swing both legs up on the wall and lie flat on your back.**

   Extend your legs up as far as possible. Extend your arms out comfortably at your sides, palms down, and relax (see Figure 10-2b).

3. **Stay in Step 2 for 2 to 10 minutes.**

218

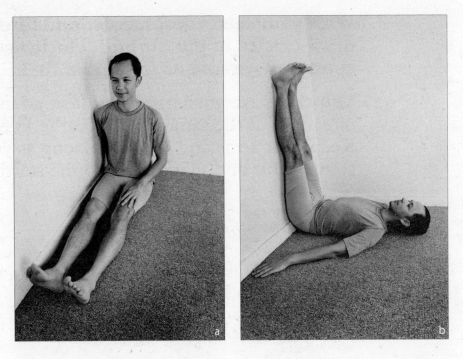

Figure 10-2:
The legs up on the wall posture.

The Happy Baby

A variation of *urdhva prasarita padasana,* Happy Baby improves circulation in the legs, arms, hips, and lower back, and has a calming effect on the nervous system. It also improves the range of motion of the ankles, toes, wrists, and fingers.

Here's how it works:

1. **Lying on your back with your knees bent and feet flat on the floor, place your arms at your sides with your palms down.**

2. **As you exhale, extend your legs and arms up vertically.**

   Keep your limbs relaxed (check out our discussion of Forgiving Limbs in Chapter 3) as you hold them up.

3. **With your feet, toes, hands, and fingers draw circles in the air both clockwise and counterclockwise as in Figure 10-3.**

You can make your hands and feet go in different directions at the same time. Breathe freely. Keep your arms and legs up as long as you feel comfortable and then return to the starting position.

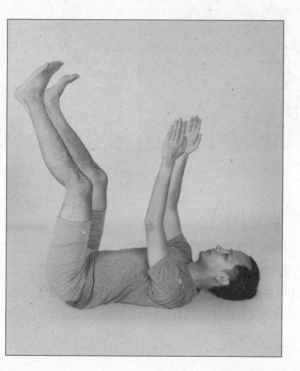

Figure 10-3:
Enjoy the freedom of movement in your ankles and wrists.

4. **Repeat Steps 2 and 3 three to five times, but don't hold the limbs up for more than a total of 5 minutes; you don't want to tire yourself out or strain your back.**

Avoid this posture if you have lower back problems.

Standing spread-legged forward bend at the wall

The standing wide-legged forward bend at the wall, which is a variation of *prasarita pada uttanasana* (described in Chapter 7), improves circulation in your head and stretches your spine and hamstrings.

Follow these easy steps:

1. **Stand with your back 2 to 3 feet from a sturdy wall, separate your feet to a comfortably wide stance, and then lean your buttocks back against the wall.**

2. **As you exhale, bend forward from the hips and hang your arms and head down.**

   If your hands touch the floor, grasp your elbows with opposite-side hands and let your forearms hang. Keep your knees soft and relax your neck and head as illustrated in Figure 10-4.

Figure 10-4:
The standing spread-legged forward bend at the wall.

3. **Stay in Step 2 for 2 to 3 minutes; use any of the Yoga breathing techniques we cover in Chapter 5.**

If you feel light-headed when doing this or any other inversion exercise, reduce the duration and increase the time gradually.

Trying a Trio of Shoulder Stands

These shoulder stands go from easiest to toughest. Each of these three shoulder stands provides common benefits: improved circulation to your legs, hips, back, neck, heart, and head. The postures all stimulate your endocrine glands and improve your lymphatic drainage, enhance elimination, and produce a calming and rejuvenating effect on your nervous system. The wall provides a useful prop for the easier two variations; when you're ready, you can then advance with confidence to *viparita karani,* the half shoulder stand.

Due to the neck's vulnerability, we recommend that you precede these postures with a dynamic (or moving) bridge posture (see Chapter 15) to prepare the neck and follow it with a short rest and then a dynamic cobra posture (see Chapter 11) to compensate.

Don't attempt any of these postures if you're pregnant; have high blood pressure or a hiatal hernia; are overweight, even moderately so; have glaucoma, diabetic retinopathy, or neck problems; or are in the first few days of your period. Also, don't use a mirrored wall, because you can injure yourself if you fall.

Half shoulder stand at the wall

This posture is a variation of *viparita karani* (see "Half

shoulder stand: Viparita karani" later in this section) and is perhaps the easiest way to pick up the half shoulder stand in a step-by-step fashion. The wall provides support as you build experience with the shoulder stand exercises.

Here's how you do it:

1. **Lie on your back with your knees bent, your feet flat on the floor, your toes just touching the base of a sturdy wall, and your arms extended along the sides of your torso with your palms down.**

2. **Place your soles up on the wall so that your bent knees form a right angle (with your thighs parallel to each other and your shins perpendicular to the wall) as in Figure 10-5a.**

   You may need to slide your buttocks closer to or farther away from the wall to get the angle just right.

3. **As you inhale, press down with your hands, push your feet to the wall, and lift your hips as high as you comfortably can as Figure 10-5b shows.**

4. **Bend your elbows and bring your hands to your lower back.**

   Press your elbows and the backs of your upper arms on the floor for support. Relax your neck (see Figure 10-5c).

Figure 10-5: Using the wall gives you support and variety.

5. **As you exhale, take one foot off the wall and extend that leg until you're looking straight up at the tip of your big toe as illustrated in Figure 10-5d.**

   You can use just one leg at a time and switch or raise both legs together. If you alternate legs, divide the time evenly between each leg.

6. **Stay in Step 4 or 5 for as long as you feel comfortable or up to 5 minutes; use the Yoga breathing techniques we recommend in Chapter 5.**

   When you want to come back down, slowly place one foot and then the other on the wall and finally lower your pelvis slowly to the floor.

Reverse half shoulder stand at the wall

The reverse half shoulder stand at the wall (see Figure 10-6b) is also a variation of *viparita karani,* which we discuss in "Half shoulder stand: Viparita karani" later in this chapter. Some people find this exercise easier than the half shoulder stand at the wall. Try them both and see which one is more comfortable for you.

To try this one, follow these steps:

1. **Lie on your back with your head toward the wall at a full arms distance from the wall with your knees bent and your feet flat on the floor at hip width as in Figure 10-6a; bring your arms back and rest your arms along the sides of your body, palms down.**

Figure 10-6: *Another way to use the wall as a prop.*

Finding the correct distance from the wall can depend on the length of your arms. Try these three different measurements: touching the wall with your fingers extended; touching with the knuckles of your fists; and touching with the backs of your hands.

2. **As you exhale, push your palms down, draw your bent knees in and up, and raise your hips to a comfortable angle of 45 to 75 degrees.**

Be sure that your legs are straight but your knees

aren't locked and that your feet are directly above your head.

3. **Bend your elbows and bring your hands to the back of your pelvis and then slide your hands up to your lower back.**

   Press your elbows and the backs of your upper arms on the floor for support.

4. **Let your toes slowly and gently touch the wall for support; relax your neck (see Figure 10-6b).**

5. **Stay in Step 4 for as long as you feel comfortable, or up to 5 minutes.**

6. **When you want to come down, ease your hips to the floor with the support of your hands and then bend your knees and lower your feet to the floor.**

Half shoulder stand: Viparita karani

You can work up to this posture by developing comfort with the half shoulder and reverse half shoulder stands at the wall (see the corresponding sections earlier in this chapter). It lets you enjoy the benefits of inversion without compressing your neck like a full shoulder stand does.

The Sanskrit word *viparita* (pronounced *vee-pah-ree-tah*) means "inverted, reversed" and *karani* (pronounced *kah-rah-nee*) means "action, process." Some authorities call this practice *sarvangasana,* meaning "all limbs posture." The word is composed of *sarva* (pronounced *sahr-vah*) and *anga* (pronounced *ahn-gah*) followed by *asana.*

When you feel you're ready, follow these steps:

1. **Lie on your back with your knees bent and your feet flat on the floor at hip width, resting your arms along the sides of your body with your palms down.**

2. **As you exhale, push your palms down, draw your bent knees in and up, and then straighten your legs as you raise your hips to a comfortable angle of 45 to 75 degrees (see Figure 10-7a).**

Figure 10-7:
The half shoulder stand.

3. **Bend your elbows and bring your hands to the back of your pelvis and then slide your hands up to your lower back.**

   Make sure your legs are straight but your knees aren't locked and your feet are directly above your head. Press your elbows and the backs of your upper arms on the floor for support. Relax your neck. Figure 11-7b shows you this portion of the posture.

4. **Stay in Step 3 for as long as you feel comfortable, or up to 5 minutes.**

5. When you want to come down, first ease your hips to the floor with the support of your hands and then bend your knees and lower your feet to the floor.

Chapter 11

Easy 'round the Bends

- -

In This Chapter

▶ Respecting your spine
▶ Introducing six back bends
▶ Checking out three side bends
▶ Venturing into four forward bends

- -

This chapter presents a variety of yogic bends. Think of them as simple extensions of the breath. Inhalation takes you naturally into a back bend, exhalation into a forward bend (for more on breath and movement, flip to Chapter 5). You can perform bending postures from many different positions — standing, kneeling, sitting, lying, or even turned upside-down (see Chapter 10). Because we cover the upright bending postures in Chapter 7 and the most popular bends for warm-up in Chapter 6, this chapter highlights the classic bending postures that you do on the floor.

Gaining a Strong Backbone (And Some Insight)

Without the spinal column, you'd never experience back pain — but then again, you couldn't walk upright either! The backbone enables you to bend forward, backward, and sideways, and it also allows you to twist. You perform all these motions every day, but you may do them unconsciously and without adequate muscular support. Yoga uses the natural movements of the spine to train the various muscles supporting it, which contributes to a healthy back and prevent back pain.

Although the spinal column's elegant curvature is well-designed for the upright position, people aren't always very clever about using it correctly. The 33 vertebrae, or backbones (24 of which comprise the flexible part of the spine), are held in place by a series of powerful muscles and ligaments that require regular exercise to maintain top working order.

Numerous muscles, arranged in several layers in the front, back, neck, and *perineum* (the area between the anus and the genitals), maintain the spine in position. When they become weak or damaged from inadequate or improper use or injury, any one of these can pull the spine out of align-

The spine as the axis of your world

According to Yoga symbolism, the spine corresponds to the axis of the universe, which is pictured as a gigantic golden mountain called *Mount Meru*. At the top of this mountain (that is, in your head) resides heaven, where all the deities are seated.

ment, leading to discomfort, pain, and inadequate nerve communication to the organs and other parts of the body, which may lead to further complications.

The spinal column is so important because it protects the spinal cord — a bundle of nerves that runs through the bony tower, your backbone. The nerves feed the trunk and limbs with information from the brain, and the brain returns the favor. If the nerve connection is severed at any point, you lose conscious control of the affected part of your body.

The spine also has psychological significance. A person of integrity and strength of character is said to "have backbone" and a coward is said to be "spineless." Because people believe that outside presentation reflects inside influences, they tend to judge a person's mental state from his bodily demeanor. If you're chronically hunched over, you signal to others that you're also inwardly collapsed. On the other hand, if you stand straight and tall, you give others the impression of self-assuredness, energy, and courage.

From a yogic point of view, the spine is the physical aspect of a subtle energetic pathway that runs from its base to the crown of the head. This pathway is known as the *central channel* or *sushumna-nadi* ("gracious conduit," pronounced *soo-shoom-nah nah-dee*). In traditional Hatha Yoga and Tantra Yoga, the awakened "serpent power," or *kundalini-shakti,* rises through this channel. When this power of pure consciousness reaches the crown of the head, you experience a sublime state of ecstasy. We say more about the central channel in Chapter 21.

Bending Over Backwards

Daily life entails a lot of forward bending: putting on a pair of pants; tying shoelaces; picking things up from the floor;

working at your computer; gardening; playing sports, and so on. A forward bend closes the front of the torso, shortens the front of the spine, and rounds the back. This closing and rounding is exaggerated by the unhealthy habit of bending forward from the waist rather than from the hip joints. Bending forward in the wrong way day in and day out can lead to spinal problems.

To experience the difference between bending from the hips and bending from the waist, sit upright in a chair with your feet flat on the floor and place your hands on the outside of your hip bones with the fingers turned inward. As you inhale, move your spine upward, lift your chest and look straight ahead. As you exhale, keep your chest lifted and bend forward: You're bending forward from the hips. Now, sit in the chair and move your hands up a few inches until they're just under your rib cage. As you exhale, bring your chin to your chest and your head down toward your thighs, bowing your spine. This bend is from the waist. Over the years, this waist-bending habit leads to what is often called a *stoop,* characterized by a sunken chest, forward-leaning head, aches and pains, and shallow breathing.

The antidote for the cumulative effects of forward bending is the regular practice of Yoga back bends, which stretch the front of the torso (and spine). Take a deep inhalation right now and notice how your torso (and spine) naturally extends during this active, opening phase of the breathing cycle, inviting you to bend backwards. Back bends are expansive, extroverted postures that can trigger powerful emotions. The major back bends usually come toward the middle of a Yoga routine so that you have plenty of time to prepare for these movements and to compensate afterwards (see Chapter 15 for more on preparation and compensation). In this section, we present some of the classic floor back bends.

To make these cobra and locust postures easier, place a small pillow or a folded blanket underneath you between your abdomen and your chest. You can move the blanket a little forward or backward to suit your needs (see Figure 11-4b later in the chapter for an illustration).

When you lie face down on the floor and raise your chest and head and use your arms in some fashion, you're doing some form of the cobra posture. When you raise just your legs, or a combination of your legs, chest, and arms, you're performing some form of the locust posture.

Move slowly and cautiously in all of the cobra and locust postures. Avoid any of the postures that cause pain in your lower back, upper back, or neck.

Cobra I

The cobra posture increases the flexibility and strength of the muscles of the arms, chest, shoulders, and back. Cobra I especially emphasizes the upper back. The cobra opens the chest, increases lung capacity, and stimulates the kidneys and the adrenals.

This first cobra posture is also called The Sphinx. It's a variation of *bhujangasana,* which we describe in the next section. To do this first version of cobra, follow these steps:

1. **Lie on your abdomen with your legs spread at hip width and the tops of your feet on the floor.**

2. **Rest your forehead on the floor and relax your shoulders; bend your elbows and place your forearms on the floor with your palms turned down and positioned near the sides of your head (see Figure 11-1a).**

Figure 11-1:
Cobra I emphasizes the upper back and is easier than cobra II.

3. **As you inhale, engage your back muscles, press your forearms against the floor, and raise your chest and head.**

   Look straight ahead, as shown in Figure 11-1b. Keep your forearms and the front of your pelvis on the floor, being mindful of relaxing your shoulders.

4. **As you exhale, lower your torso and head slowly back to the floor.**

5. **Repeat Steps 3 and 4 three times and then stay in Step 3 (the last raised position) for 6 to 8 breaths.**

If you have lower back problems, separate your legs wider than your hips and let your heels turn out and your toes turn in.

Cobra II: Bhujangasana

This posture rewards you with most of the same benefits as cobra I, which we describe in the preceding section. In addition, cobra II emphasizes flexibility in your lower back.

The following steps walk you through cobra II:

1. **Lie on your abdomen with your legs spread at hip width and the tops of your feet on the floor.**

2. **Bend your elbows and place your palms on the**

floor with your thumbs near your armpits.

Rest your forehead on the floor and relax your shoulders, as shown in Figure 11-2a.

Figure 11-2:
Cobra II emphasizes flexibility in the lower back.

3. **As you inhale, press your palms against the floor, engage your back muscles, and raise your chest and head.**

   Look straight ahead (see Figure 11-2b). Keep the top front of your pelvis on the floor and your shoulders relaxed. Unless you're very flexible, keep your elbows slightly bent.

4. **As you exhale, lower your torso and head slowly back to the floor.**

5. **Repeat Steps 3 and 4 three times and then stay in Step 3 (the last raised position) for 6 to 8 breaths.**

Note: In the *classic* (traditionally taught) posture, the inner legs are joined and the knees are straight. The head is in alignment with the spine and the eyes look forward. The palms are on the floor close to the sides of the torso near the navel, the elbows are slightly bent and the shoulders relaxed.

If you move your hands farther forward, the cobra is less difficult; if you move your hands farther back you increase the difficulty.

The Sanskrit word *bhujangasana* is composed of *bhujanga* (pronounced *bhooj-ahng-gah*), meaning "serpent," and *asana,* or "posture."

Cobra III

Cobra III, which is another version of the classic *bhujangasana,* is unique because it doesn't ask you to place your hands on the floor. The emphasis is on strengthening both the lower and upper back.

Try out cobra III by following these steps:

1. **Lie on your abdomen with your legs spread at hip width and the tops of your feet on the floor; rest your forehead on the floor.**

2. **Extend your arms back along the sides of your torso with your palms on the floor as Figure 11-3a illustrates.**

Figure 11-3:
Cobra III strengthens the lower and upper back and the neck.

3. **As you inhale, raise your chest and head and sweep your arms like wings out to the sides and then all the way forward.**

   Keep your legs on the floor, as shown in Figure 11-3b.

4. **As you exhale, sweep your arms back and lower your torso and your head slowly to the floor.**

5. **Repeat Steps 3 and 4 three times and then stay in Step 3 (the last raised position) for 6 to 8 breaths.**

Locust I: Shalabhasana

The locust posture strengthens the entire torso including the lower back and the neck. In addition, it strengthens the buttocks and the legs and improves digestion and elimination.

To try this first locust posture, follow these steps:

1. **Lie on your abdomen with your legs spread at hip width and the tops of your feet on the floor; rest your forehead on the floor.**

2. **Extend your arms along the sides of your torso with your palms on the floor.**

3. **As you inhale, raise your chest, head, and one leg up and away from the floor as high as is**

To clench or not to clench: That is the question

An ongoing controversy in the Yoga world is "Should the buttocks be firm or soft in the cobra?" The traditional instruction is to firm the buttocks. However, the work of New Zealand-born physiotherapist Robin McKenzie has revolutionized back care — and ideas about back bends. In his own version of the cobra, called *The McKenzie Technique,* McKenzie suggests that the buttocks be soft to facilitate the healing of numerous lower back ailments. Try the cobra both ways, with the buttocks firm or soft, and see which feels best to you. ***Note:*** This discussion applies to cobra only; in all the locust postures, the buttocks are usually tight.

---

comfortable for you (see Figure 11-4a).

Figure 11-4:
Raise your chest, head, and leg on an inhale, using a blanket if necessary.

Consider trying this posture with blankets for more personal comfort. Figure 11-4b shows you the basic blanket positioning, though you can shift it as necessary.

4. **As you exhale, lower your chest, head, and leg together slowly to the floor and repeat Steps 3 and 4 with the other leg.**

5. **Repeat Steps 3 and 4 three times and then stay in Step 3 (the last raised position) for 6 to 8 breaths.**

You can increase the level of difficulty by raising both legs at the same time in Step 3.

Note: In the classic posture, the inner legs are joined, the knees are straight.

Locust II

This posture, which is another variation of *shalabhasana,* also teaches the two sides of the body how to work independently of one another. Many back problems are due to imbalances in the muscle system on each side of the spine. Health professionals often call this situation an *asymmetrical problem.* Locust II helps bring your back into symmetry

238

again and also improves your coordination.

The following steps get you on the road to enjoying these benefits:

1. **Lie on your abdomen with your legs spread at hip width and the tops of your feet on the floor; rest your forehead on the floor.**

2. **Extend your right arm forward with your palm resting on the floor; bring your left arm back along the left side of your torso, with the back of your hand on the floor as shown in Figure 11-5a.**

Figure 11-5:
This posture balances the muscles on each side of your back.

3. **As you inhale, slowly raise your chest, head, right arm, and left leg up and away from the floor as high as is comfortable for you.**

   Try to keep the upper right arm and ear in alignment, and raise your left foot and right hand to the same height above the floor (see Figure 11-5b).

4. **As you exhale, lower your right arm, chest, head, and left leg slowly to the floor at the same time.**

5. **Repeat Steps 3 and 4 three times and then stay in Step 3 for 6 to 8 breaths.**

6. **Repeat Steps 1 through 5 with opposite pairs (left arm and right leg).**

Locust II features some interesting biomechanics. When you raise the chest and the right arm, you strengthen the right side of your upper back. When you raise the left leg, you strengthen the right side of your lower back. So even though this posture uses opposite arms and legs, it strengthens one side of the upper and lower back at a time.

Avoid locust variations that lift just the legs. Lifting the legs alone increases interabdominal and chest pressure, heart rate, and tension in the neck.

Locust III: Superman posture

This posture, a further variation of *shalabhasana,* gets its name from the image of Superman flying through the air at warp speed, with his arms extended out in front leading the way. It's the most strenuous back bend because fully extending your arms and legs as shown in Figure 11-6 puts quite a load on your entire back. Use this pose only after you're comfortable with locust I and II.

This posture is physically challenging. Don't attempt it if you're having back or neck problems.

If you're ready and able, try the following steps:

1. **Lie on your abdomen with your legs spread at hip width and the tops of your feet on the floor; extend your arms back along the sides of your torso with your palms on the floor and rest your forehead on the floor (see Figure 11-6a).**

Figure 11-6:
Make sure you're ready for this "super" posture.

2. **As you inhale, raise your chest, legs, and head and sweep your arms like wings out to the sides and then all the way forward as Figure 11-6b illustrates.**

In the beginning, try sweeping your arms only halfway forward in a *T* position; it allows your back muscles to gradually become accustomed to the posture's physical demands.

3. **As you exhale, sweep your arms back and lower your torso, legs, and head slowly to the floor at the same time.**

4. **Repeat Steps 2 and 3 three times and then stay in Step 2 (the last raised position) for 6 to 8 breaths.**

Bending from Side to Side

The spinal column can move in four basic ways: forward *(flexion)*, backward *(extension)*, sideways *(lateral flexion)*, and twist *(rotation)*. The side bend is often the least practiced in Yoga. This missed opportunity is unfortunate because side bends help to stretch and tone the muscles along the sides of the abdomen, rib cage, and spine, keeping your waist trim, your breathing full, and your spine supple.

A true side bend fully contracts one side of the body while expanding the other. To experience the effects of a side bend right now, simply lean over to your right (or left) side as you exhale and reach the same-side arm downward. To realize the full effect of the stretch, reach the opposite-side arm up toward the ceiling. In this section, we cover some safe, creative ways to use side bends on the floor.

Seated side bend

This seated side bend is a great way to ease into the position if you're not used to bending from side to side. Just follow these steps:

1. **Sit comfortably in a simple cross-legged position.**

   Place your right palm on the floor, near your right hip. Check out Chapter 6 for some appropriate seated positions.

2. **As you inhale, raise your left arm out to the side and up above your head beside your left ear.**

3. **As you exhale, slide your right hand across the floor out to the right, letting your torso, head, and left arm follow as you bend to the right as Figure 11-7 shows.**

   Don't let your buttocks come off the floor as you bend.

Figure 11-7:
Slide your hand across the floor as you bend.

4. **As you inhale, return to the upright position (as you were at the start of Step 2).**

5. **Repeat Steps 2 through 4 three times and then stay in the bent position (Step 3) for 6 to 8 breaths.**

6. **Repeat Steps 1 through 5 on the other side.**

All-fours side bend

Many people with back or hip problems have a hard time sitting upright on the floor. The all-fours position gives the spine more freedom and is an easier side bend from the floor. Follow these steps to enjoy the benefits:

1. **Start on your hands and knees, with your knees below your hips and your hands below your shoulders with your palms on the floor.**

243

Straighten your elbows, but don't lock them. Look straight ahead.

2. **As you exhale, bend your head and torso sideways to the right and look toward your tailbone (see Figure 11-8).**

3. **As you inhale, return to the starting position in Step 1.**

4. **Repeat Steps 2 and 3 three times and then stay in Step 2 for 6 to 8 breaths.**

5. **Repeat Steps 2 through 4 on the other side.**

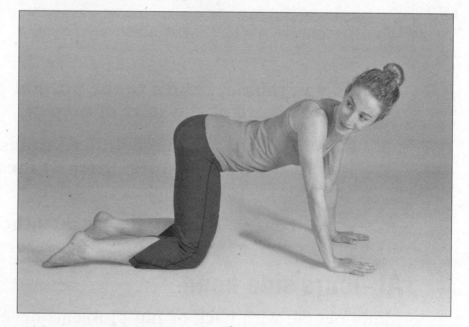

Figure 11-8:
Look back as you bend.

Folded side bend

The Sanskrit word *bala* (pronounced *bah-lah*) means "child." This practice was inspired by a baby's folded position in the womb. The benefits of this side bend, which is a variation of *balasana,* the child's posture (covered in

244

Chapter 15), are the same as for the seated side bend.

The following steps show you how it works:

1. **Sit on your heels with your toes pointing back and fold forward by laying your abdomen on your thighs and your head on the floor.**

   Extend your arms forward with your palms on the floor as in Figure 11-9a.

Figure 11-9:
Wait a few moments before you stretch farther on each side.

2. **As you exhale, stay in the folded position and slide your upper torso, head, arms, and hands to the right as far as possible, as shown in Figure 11-9b.**

   Wait for a few seconds and again, with another exhalation, slide farther to the right if you can do so without straining.

3. **Return to center and repeat the sequence to the left side, staying in Step 2 for 6 to 8 breaths on each side.**

Bending Forward

Of all the ways the human torso (and spine) can move, bending forward is the maneuver folks most commonly use. A tucked or fetal position is inherently comforting to most people, perhaps because they spend their first nine months positioned like that in their mothers' wombs.

Forward bends are usually a good way to begin any movement routine (unless you're dealing with spinal disc injuries or certain other back problems). Though back bends are the lively extroverts of the *asana* family, forward bends are the retiring introverts; they're always performed with an exhalation — the passive, contracting phase of the breathing cycle.

Constantly bending forward from the waist tends to put stress on the lower back and neck. Yogic forward bends call for movement from the hip joints, a switch that can help you maintain a healthy, stress-free spine as you correct the poor forward-bending habits we discuss earlier in this chapter.

 Be very careful of all the seated forward bends if you have disc-related back problems.

If you have a problem sitting upright on the floor in the seated forward bend or in any of the following forward bending postures, raise your hips with folded blankets or firm pillows, as shown in Figure 11-10c.

Seated forward bend: Pashcimottanasana

The seated forward bend intensely stretches the entire back side of the body, including the back of the spine and legs. It also tones the muscles and organs of the abdomen and creates a calming and quieting effect.

To enjoy these benefits, try the following:

1. **Sit on the floor with your legs at hip width and comfortably stretched out in front of you.**

Bring your back up nice and tall and place your palms down on the floor near your thighs.

2. **As you inhale, raise your arms forward and up overhead until they're beside your ears as shown in Figure 11-10a.**

   Keep your arms and legs soft and slightly bent in Forgiving Limbs, which we describe in Chapter 3.

3. **As you exhale, bend forward from the hips; bring your hands, chest, and head toward your legs.**

   Rest your hands on the floor, your thighs, knees, shins, or feet. If your head isn't close to your knees, bend your knees more until you feel your back stretching (see Figure 11-10b).

4. **Repeat Steps 2 and 3 three times and then stay folded (Step 3) for 6 to 8 breaths.**

Figure 11-10:
If your head isn't close to your knees, bend your knees more.

Note: In the classic posture, the inner legs are joined, the knees are straight, and the ankles are extended so that the toes point up. The chin rests on the chest, the hands hold the sides of the feet, the back is extended forward, and the forehead is pressed against the legs.

In Sanskrit, *pashcimottanasana* (pronounced *pash-chee-moh-tah-nah-sah-nah*) translates to the "extension of the West posture." In yogic jargon, the West refers to the back, and the East stands for the front. The symbolism refers to both the physical and psychological effects of this posture: It stretches the back of the body, especially the back of the spine and legs, and just as the sun sets in the West, the "light" of your consciousness draws inward as you fold upon yourself.

Head-to-knee posture: Janushirshasana

The head-to-knee posture keeps your spine supple, stimulates the abdominal organs, and stretches your back, especially on the side of the extended leg. It also activates the central channel *(sushumna-nadi)*. As we explain in Chapter 5, the *central channel* is the pathway for the awakened energy of pure consciousness (called *kundalini-shakti*), which leads to ecstasy and spiritual liberation.

Follow these steps to achieve this posture:

1. **Sit on the floor with your legs stretched out in front of you and then bend your left knee and bring your left heel toward your right groin.**

2. **Rest your bent left knee on the floor (but don't force it down) and place the sole of your left foot on the inside of your right thigh.**

   The toes of the left foot point toward the right knee.

3. **Bring your back up nice and tall; as you inhale, raise your arms forward and up overhead until they're beside your ears as Figure 11-11a shows.**

Keep your arms and the right leg soft and slightly bent in Forgiving Limbs, which we describe in Chapter 3.

Figure 11-11:
The head-to-knee posture.

4. **As you exhale, bend forward from the hips, bringing your hands, chest and head toward your right leg.**

Rest your hands on the floor or your thigh, knee, shin, or foot. If your head isn't close to your right knee, bend your knee more until you feel your back stretching on the right side (see Figure 11-11b).

5. **Repeat Steps 3 and 4 three times and then stay in Step 4 (the final forward bend) for 6 to 8 breaths.**

6. **Repeat Steps 1 through 4 on the opposite side.**

Keep your back muscles as relaxed as possible.

The Sanskrit word *janu* (pronounced *jah-noo*) means "knee," and *shirsha* (pronounced *sheer-shah*) means "head."

Volcano: Mahamudra

Ancient Hatha Yoga texts give high praise to the volcano posture. It strengthens the back, stretches the legs, and opens the hips and chest. This posture is unique in that it has qualities of both a forward bend and a back bend. When used with special locks *(bandhas)* that contain and channel energy in the torso, this technique has both cleansing and healing effects.

Here's how to do it:

1. **Sitting on the floor with your legs stretched out in front of you, bend your left knee and bring your left foot toward your right groin.**

2. **Rest your bent left knee on the floor to the left (but don't force it down), and place the sole of your left foot on the inside of your right thigh with your heel in your groin.**

   The toes of the left foot point toward the right knee.

3. **Bring your back up nice and tall; as you inhale, raise your arms forward and up overhead until they're beside your ears.**

   Keep your arms and the right leg soft and slightly bent in Forgiving Limbs, as we describe in Chapter 3. Refer to Figure 11-11a in the preceding section if necessary.

250

4. **As you exhale, bend forward from the hips, lift your chest forward, and extend your back without letting it round.**

   Place your hands on the right knee, shin, or toes and look straight ahead (see Figure 11-12).

5. **Repeat Steps 3 and 4 three times and then stay in Step 4 for 6 to 8 breaths.**

6. **Repeat the same sequence on the opposite side.**

Note: In the classic posture, the front leg and the arms are straight, and the hands are holding the toes of the front leg. The back is extended and the chin is pressed on the chest. The abdominal muscles are pulled up into the abdominal cavity and the anal sphincter is tightened.

The Sanskrit term *mahamudra* (pronounced *mah-hah-mood-rah*) means literally "great seal." Here it applies to a Yoga posture, but in other contexts, *mahamudra* is a mental exercise that allows your mind to flow out into the open sky. Try combining this inner "attitude" with the physical pose.

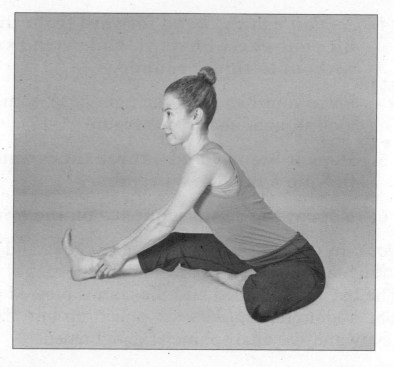

Figure 11-12:
The volcano is a great, all-inclusive posture.

Spread-legged forward bend: Upavishta konasana

The spread-legged forward bend stretches the backs and insides of the legs (hamstrings and adductors) and increases the flexibility of the spine and hip joints. It improves circulation to the entire pelvic region, tones the abdomen, and has a calming effect on the nervous system. Note, though, that muscle density may make this posture difficult for most men. If you want to give it a try, check out the following steps:

1. **Sit on the floor, with your legs straight and spread wide apart (but not more than 90 degrees).**

   Because this posture is challenging, give yourself an advantage by pulling the flesh of the buttocks (you may know them as "cheeks") out from under the *sits bones* (the bones directly under that flesh; they're also known as the *ischial tuberosities*) and bending your knees slightly. Alternatively, sit on some folded blankets.

2. **As you inhale, raise your arms forward and up overhead until they're beside your ears.**

   Keep your elbows soft and your legs slightly bent in Forgiving Limbs, as we describe in Chapter 3. Bring your back up nice and tall (see Figure 11-13a).

Figure 11-13:
The spread-legged forward bend.

3. **As you exhale, bend forward from the hips and bring your hands, chest, and head toward the floor.**

   Rest your extended arms and hands palms down on the floor. If you have the flexibility, place your forehead on the floor as well as shown in Figure 11-13b.

4. **Repeat Steps 2 and 3 three times and then stay in Step 3 (the folded position) for 6 to 8 breaths.**

Note: In the classic posture, the legs are straight with the toes vertical, the chin and chest are on the floor, and the arms are extended forward with the palms joined.

The spread-legged forward bend is also called the *lifetime posture* because it can take a whole lifetime to master. But don't worry if you don't quite reach mastery. According to Yoga's outlook, if you don't master the pose in this lifetime, you can try again in the next lifetime.

 The Sanskrit term *upavishta* (pronounced *oopah-vish-tah*) means "seated" and *kona* (pronounced *koh-nah*) means "angle."

Chapter 12

Several Twists on the Yoga Twist

Imagine you're cleaning up the kitchen with a wet sponge. After mopping up some spills the sponge gets dirty. You hold it under the kitchen faucet, turn on the water, and squeeze out the dirty water. As you release the pressure on the sponge, it sucks up some clean water. You're ready to start again.

This sponge analogy helps to visualize how yogic twists work on the spine. The pulpy pads between the individual bones, called the *intervertebral discs* have no direct blood supply of their own after about age 20, so they depend on your everyday movements to help them wring out the accumulated wastes and, in turn, soak up a fresh supply of blood and other reviving fluids. This process is called *imbibation*. Over time, if your discs aren't continually squeezed and soaked, they tend to harden and dry out, like a sponge left unused for a few days. Consequently, your spine stiffens up and shrinks.

Twists are an important component of any Yoga practice. They clean out the discs and help keep them firm and supple; massage the internal organs, such as your intestines and kidneys; stoke the inner fire of digestion; and stretch and strengthen the muscles of your back and abdomen.

This chapter features seated twists, which emphasize the upper spine, and reclining twists, which emphasize the lower spine. For standing twists, see Chapter 8.

 Approach all twists with caution if you're suffering from disc problems anywhere in your spine. Consult your physician, chiropractor, or physical therapist or work with a reputable Yoga therapist after you have a diagnosis.

Trying Simple Upright Twists

When thinking about the human body and mind, people often associate the word *twist* with pain or something undesirable. For example, people say things like, "She twisted her ankle," "He has a twisted mind," or "She accused him of twisting her words." But twisting isn't all bad. Ropes get their strength from the twisted strands that comprise them. Yogic twisting postures have the same positive effect. When done properly, they bring strength to your body, especially to the weak spots (notably the lower back). True enough, twisting is part of your everyday movements. But unless your muscles are well trained, you can easily injure yourself. The exercises in this section can help you get your back in tip-top shape as you look forward to enjoyment and enlightenment along the way.

Easy chair twist

This seated posture is an excellent way for a beginner to achieve a good twist safely before moving on to more complex methods of twisting. And, you can use this simple, effective posture to liberate your spine while at the office without drawing too much attention to yourself. Your spine will thank you!

Twist mainly from your shoulders; the head and neck come along for the ride.

1. **Sit sideways on a chair with the chair back to your left, your feet flat on the floor, and your heels directly below your knees.**

2. **Exhale, turn to the left, and hold the sides of the chair back with your hands.**

3. **As you inhale, extend or lift your spine upward.**

4. **As you exhale, twist your torso and head farther to the left as in Figure 12-1.**

5. **Repeat Steps 1 through 4, gradually twisting farther with each exhalation, for 3 breaths (don't force it) and then hold the twist for 6 to 8 breaths.**

6. **Repeat Steps 1 through 5 on the opposite side.**

If your feet aren't comfortably on the floor for the easy chair twist, elevate them with a folded blanket or a phone book.

Figure 12-1:
Easy chair twist.

Easy sitting twist

After you can twist comfortably while seated on a chair (see the preceding section), you can transfer your newly gained skill to the floor and try the following exercise. Its effect is similar to that of the easy chair twist, and it fits nicely into a regular Yoga practice, a large part of which may be done on the floor.

1. **Sit on the floor with your legs in a simple cross-legged position and extend your spine upward, nice and tall.**

2. **Place your left hand palm down on top of your right knee.**

3. **Place your right hand palm down on the floor behind your right hip to prop yourself up.**

4. **As you inhale, extend your spine upward.**

5. **As you exhale, twist your torso and head to the right (see Figure 12-2).**

Figure 12-2:
The easy sitting twist.

6. **Repeat Steps 4 and 5 for 3 breaths, gradually twisting farther with each exhalation (don't force it), and then hold the twist for 6 to 8 breaths.**

7. **Repeat Steps 1 through 6 on the opposite side.**

If you have difficulty sitting upright in this seated twist, use blankets or pillows to make your hips even with your knees.

The sage twist

The easy chair twist and the easy sitting twist we cover in the preceding sections are the simplest yogic twists. By changing the position of your legs, you can alter the level

259

of difficulty and also enhance the overall benefit. The sage twist does just that to give you extra rewards for your investment.

1. **Sit on the floor with both legs extended forward; bend your right knee and place your right foot on the floor just inside your left thigh, with your toes facing forward.**

2. **Place your right hand, palm down, on the floor behind you; wrap the palm of your left hand around the side of your right knee.**

3. **As you inhale, extend or lift your spine upward.**

4. **As you exhale, twist your torso and head to the right as shown in Figure 12-3.**

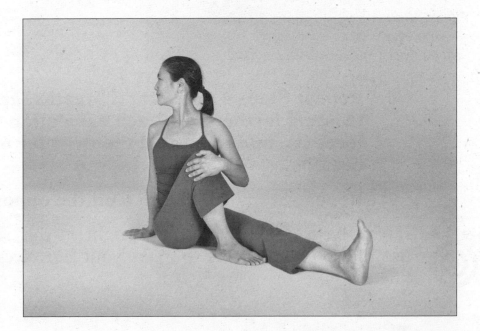

Figure 12-3:
Beginners can enjoy benefits from this sage twist variation.

5. **Repeat Steps 3 and 4, gradually twisting farther with each exhalation, for 3 breaths (don't force it) and then hold the twist for 6 to 8 breaths.**

6. Repeat Steps 1 through 5 on the opposite side.

If you have difficulty sitting upright in this seated twist, sit on blankets or pillows until your hips are even with your knees.

This posture is a variation of the classic posture called *maricy-asana*. The Sanskrit word *marici* (pronounced *mah-ree-chee*) means "ray of light" and is the name of an ancient sage.

Twisting While Reclining

The twists in the preceding section all require you to sit upright, but the remaining exercises in this chapter call for you to lie down — with a (literal) twist. In the twists described in this section, you harvest all kinds of benefits, including a delicious feeling of release in your spine.

Bent leg supine twist

The bent supine twist is a variation of the classic posture known as *parivartanasana*. The Sanskrit word *parivartana* (pronounced *pah-ree-vahr-tah-nah*) means "turning."

This posture has a calming effect on the lower back. Here's how you do it:

1. **Lie on your back with your knees bent and feet on the floor at hip width and extend your arms out from your sides like a *T* (in line with the top of your shoulders) with your palms down.**

2. **As you exhale, slowly lower your bent legs to the right side while turning your head to the left (see Figure 12-4).**

   Keep your head on the floor.

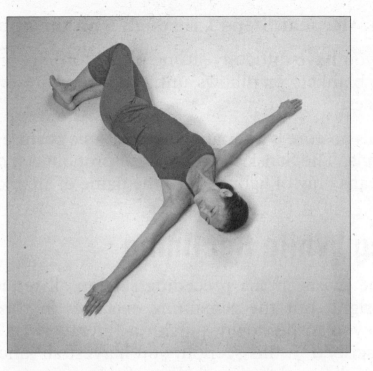

Figure 12-4:
Turn your head the opposite direction of your legs.

3. As you inhale, bring your bent knees back to the middle.

4. As you exhale, slowly lower your bent knees to the left while turning your head to the right.

5. Repeat Steps 1 through 4, alternating three times slowly on each side, and then hold one last twist on each side for 6 to 8 breaths.

The Swiss army knife

This posture, a variation of the classic *jathara parivritti,* tones the abdominal organs and intestines and stretches the lower back and hips. *Jathara parivritti* (pronounced *jat-hah-rah pah-ree-vree-tee*) means "belly twisting." Just follow these steps:

1. Lie flat on the floor with your legs straight down and extend your arms out from your

262

sides like a *T* (in line with the top of your shoulders) with your palms up.

2. Bend your right knee and draw your thigh into your abdomen.

3. As you exhale, slowly lower your bent right leg to the left side and extend it out a comfortable distance.

4. Extend your left arm on the floor along the left side of your head (palm up), and then turn your head to the right as shown in Figure 12-5.

   Keep your head on the floor and try to visualize lines of energy going out through your arms and legs.

5. Follow Steps 1 through 4 and then relax and stay in Step 4 for 6 to 8 breaths.

6. Repeat Steps 1 through 5 on the opposite side.

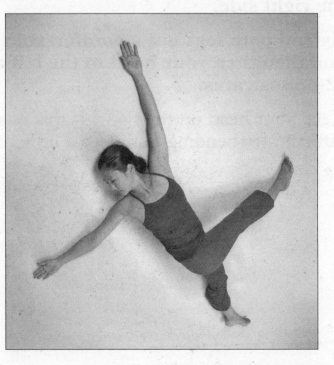

Figure 12-5:
Extend your arm and turn your head the opposite way.

Extended legs supine twist: Jathara parivritti

If you enjoy practicing the Swiss army knife (see the preceding section), you're likely to enjoy this slightly more demanding exercise. This variation of *jathara parivritti* gives you the same benefits as the Swiss army knife but creates an even more pronounced stretch of the lower back and hips. And, of course, stretching is good for your muscles and your spine. The following steps show you how it works:

1. **Lie on your back with your knees bent and feet on the floor at hip width and extend your arms out from your sides like a *T* in line with the top of your shoulders with palms down.**

2. **Bend your knees and draw both your thighs into your abdomen.**

3. **As you exhale, slowly lower your bent legs to the right side.**

4. **Extend both legs out a comfortable distance and then turn your head to the left as Figure 12-6 illustrates.**

   Keep your head on the floor. If this posture is difficult, try bending both legs a little more.

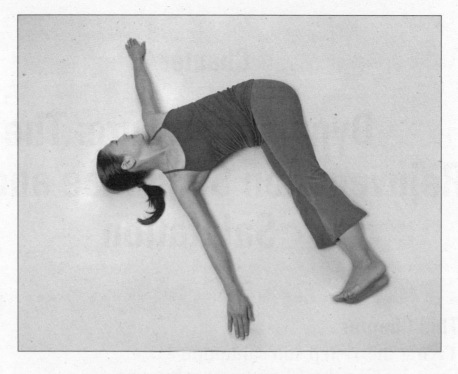

Figure 12-6:
Keep your head on the floor as you turn it and extend your legs.

5. **Follow Steps 1 through 4 and then relax and stay in Step 4 for 6 to 8 breaths.**

6. **Repeat Steps 1 through 5 on the opposite side.**

Note: In the *classic* (traditionally taught) version of this posture, the knees are straight and the joined legs are resting on the floor. The arms are straight and extended to the sides at right angles to the torso. The hand on the same side of the extended legs holds the top foot.

Chapter 13

Dynamic Posture: The Rejuvenation Sequence and Sun Salutation

The sun has long captured humanity's attention for its life-giving power. Sun worship is one of humankind's first and most natural forms of spiritual expression: Just think of the Sumerians, Egyptians, and Mayans. But nowhere has this homage to the solar spirit been as well preserved as in India's 10,000-year-old civilization, where to this day millions of people pay respects to the sun as a part of their daily rituals.

You don't have to be a sun worshiper, though, to benefit from Yoga's sun salutation (*surya namaskara,* pronounced *soor-yah nah-mahs-kah-rah*). This exercise — a special sequence of postures — is considered so profound many people use it on its own.

The sun salutation helps you remember the Yogic idea that your body is condensed sunlight. The saluting gesture, called *namaskara mudra* in Sanskrit (pronounced *nah-mahs-kah-rah mood-rah*), is a salute to the highest aspect within yourself — the spirit.

The actual technique for and number of steps in the sun salutation vary somewhat among the different Yoga schools and organizations. Of course, each school claims to practice the original sun salutation. In this chapter, we focus on the best-known form of sun salutation — a 12-step sequence introduced to America in the early 1950s by the late Swami Vishnu Devananda, a disciple of the great Swami Shivananda of Rishikesh, India. First, though, we introduce a modified 7-step version you do from a kneeling position; it's ideally suited for those who have yet to develop enough flexibility, muscle strength, and fitness for the 12-step version.

The dawn of the sun salutation

No one knows how old the sun salutation is, but at the beginning of the 20th century, the Raja of Oudh, representing a small state in Northern India, encouraged all his subjects to learn and practice this exercise sequence. He personally practiced the sun salutation for health and happiness.

Warming up for the Sun: Rejuvenating in 9 Steps

Do you need a more user-friendly version of the sun salutation? Do you have a hard time kneeling (as required in the 7-step sun salutation later in this chapter) or stepping through (as required in the 12-step sun salutation later in this chapter)? Then try the 9-step rejuvenation sequence direct from California, using the focus breathing technique from Chapter 5:

1. **Stand in the mountain posture with your feet at hip width and arms at your sides (see Figure 13-1a).**

2. **As you inhale, slowly raise your arms out from the sides and up overhead (see Figure 13-1b) and then pause.**

3. **As you exhale, bend forward from the waist and bring your head toward your knees and your hands forward and down toward the floor in the standing forward bend (see Figure 13-1c).**

   Keep your arms and legs soft (see Chapter 3 for an explanation of Forgiving Limbs). Then pause.

4. **Bend your knees quite a bit and as you inhale, sweep your arms out from the sides, but only come halfway up with your arms in a *T* (half forward bend), as shown in Figure 13-1d.**

   Then pause briefly.

5. **As you exhale, fold all the way down again and hang your arms in the standing forward bend (see Figure 13-1e).**

6. **As you inhale, sweep your arms from the sides like wings and bring your torso all the way up again, standing with your arms overhead in the standing arm raise (see Figure 13-1f).**

7. **As you exhale, bend your knees and squat halfway to the floor.**

   Soften your arms but keep them overhead; look straight ahead (see Figure 13-1g).

Inhale → Exhale →

Inhale → Exhale → Inhale →

Figure 13-1:
The 9-step rejuvenation sequence.

Exhale → Inhale → Exhale →

8. **As you inhale, bring your torso all the way up again, standing with your arms overhead in the standing arm raise (see Figure 13-1h).**

9. **As you exhale, bring your arms back to your sides as in Step 1 (see Figure 13-1i).**

Repeat the entire sequence 6 to 8 times slowly.

269

To make it harder on the last round, stay for 6 to 8 breaths in the half forward bend (Step 4), the standing forward bend (Step 5), and the half squat or half chair (Step 8).

To make it much harder, do the entire sequence standing on your toes.

Gliding Through the 7-Step Kneeling Salutation

If you aren't quite ready to tackle the 12-step sun salutation, the following 7-step variation can give you many benefits and also help you get in shape for the standing variety. Use focus, chest-to-belly, or belly-to-chest breathing techniques from Chapter 5 and follow these steps.

Just follow your breath — inhale when you're opening, exhale when you're folding. Move slowly, pausing after each inhalation and exhalation.

1. **Sit on your heels in a bent-knee position, bring your back up nice and tall, and place your palms together in the prayer position with the thumbs touching the sternum (breastbone) in the middle of your chest (see Figure 13-2a).**

2. **As you inhale, open your palms and slightly raise your arms forward and then up and overhead; raise your buttocks away from your heels, arch your back, and look up at the ceiling as illustrated in Figure 13-2b.**

3. **As you exhale, bend forward slowly from the hips, placing your palms, forearms, and then your forehead on the floor and pause relaxing your hip as Figure 13-2c shows.**

4. **Slide your hands forward on the floor until your arms are extended and then slide your chest forward, bending your elbows slightly, and arch up into cobra II as shown in Figure 13-2d.**

   Flip to Chapter 11 for instructions on cobra II.

Figure 13-2:
The 7-step
sun
salutation.

5. **As you exhale, turn your toes under, raise your hips up, extend your legs, and bring your chest down keeping both hands on the floor for the downward-facing dog (see Figure 13-2e).**

6. **As you inhale, bend your knees to the floor and look straight ahead like in Figure 13-2f.**

7. **As you exhale, sit back on your heels and return your hands to the saluting position as in Step 1 (Figure 13-2g).**

Repeat the entire sequence 3 to 12 times.

Shedding light on the benefits of sun saluting

Respected for its excellent effects, the sun salutation reputedly provides an array of benefits, including the following:

✔ Stretching your spine and strengthening the muscles that support it

✔ Strengthening and stretching your arms and legs

✔ Improving your posture, coordination, and endurance

✔ Complementing the delicate balance between muscle tension and muscle relaxation

✔ Linking body, breath, and mind

✔ Granting (in most of its forms) aerobic benefits

✔ Improving your lung function and the delivery of oxygen to your muscles (including the heart)

✔ Working well (with modifications) for people of all ages, from children to seniors

The Yoga masters claim that the sun salutation has deeper psychological and spiritual implications because it stimulates subtle vital energies leading to states of higher awareness. No wonder so many Yoga videos on the market today include the sun salutation!

If you are not able to sit on your heels in Steps 1 and 7, simply keep your palms in prayer position and stand on your knees instead. You can also fold a blanket under your knees for comfort.

 If you find this 7-step salutation too difficult for you, head to the following section and try Steps 1 through 3 only of the 12-step version until you're ready to do more.

Advancing to the 12-Step Sun Salutation

To enjoy the greatest benefit from this sequence (as well as all your Yoga postures), execute each part with full participation of your mind. When you stand, really stand; plant your feet firmly on the ground. When you bend or stretch, bend or stretch with complete attention. Your mind makes your practice not only elegant but also potent. Use any of the Yoga breathing techniques from Chapter 5 and follow these steps:

1. **Start in a standing position with your feet at hip width and place your palms together in the prayer position with your thumbs touching the *sternum* (breastbone) in the middle of your chest as Figure 13-3a illustrates.**

2. **As you inhale, open your palms slightly and raise your arms forward and up and overhead; arch your back and look up at the ceiling (see Figure 13-3b).**

3. **As you exhale, bend forward from the hips, soften your knees (as in Forgiving Limbs, covered in Chapter 3), and place your hands on**

the floor; bring your head as close as possible to your legs as shown in Figure 13-3c.

4. **As you inhale, bend your left knee and step your right foot back into a lunge.**

   Make sure that your left knee is directly over your ankle and your thigh is parallel to the floor, so that your knee forms a right angle. Look straight ahead; Figure 13-3d gives you a visual of this step.

5. **As you exhale, step your left foot back beside the right and hold a push-up position; if your arms tire, bend your knees to the floor and pause on your hands and knees (see Figure 13-3e).**

6. **Inhale and then as you exhale, lower your knees (from the push-up), chest, and chin to the floor, keeping your buttocks up in the air as illustrated in Figure 13-3f.**

7. **As you inhale, slide your chest forward along the floor and then arch back into cobra II as in Figure 13-3g.**

8. **As you exhale, turn your toes under, raise your hips up, extend your legs, and bring your chest down, keeping both hands on the floor as shown in Figure 13-3h.**

9. **As you inhale, step your right foot forward between your hands and look straight ahead (see Figure 13-3i).**

10. **As you exhale, step your left foot forward, parallel to and even with the right; soften your knees and fold into a forward bend as in Step 3 and Figure 13-3j.**

11. **As you inhale, raise your arms either forward and up overhead from the front, or out and up from the sides like wings, and then arch back and look up, as in Step 2 as Figure 13-3k indicates.**

If you have back problems, lifting up from the forward bend with your arms to the front or sides may cause you some discomfort. If so, you can try the roll up: Keep your chin on your chest and roll up, stacking the vertebrae one at a time, with your arms hanging at your sides, head coming up last. When you're fully upright, bring the arms forward, up, and overhead from the front, arch your back just a little, and look up.

12. **As you exhale, return your hands to the prayer position as in Step 1 and Figure 13-3l.**

Repeat the entire sequence 3 to 12 times. First lead with the right foot, and then alternate with the left foot, for an equal number of repetitions (each side counts as half a sequence).

If you're ready for greater challenges, consider the advanced sun salutations in *Power Yoga For Dummies* by Doug Swenson (Wiley) from the Ashtanga Yoga system, or check the Internet for the Iyengar sun salutation or various "flow" sequences.

Figure 13-3:
The 12-step sun salutation.

Chapter 14

A Recommended Beginners' Routine for Men and Women

• •

In This Chapter

▶ Keeping current on basic Yoga principles

▶ Presenting a basic Yoga routine for beginners

• •

The Yoga routine in this chapter is a tried-and-true sequence from my (Larry's) Larry Payne's Prime of Life
Yoga and is an excellent way for a beginner to get started.
Taught around the world, this sequence has helped thousands of people — including the staff at the J. Paul Getty
Museum in Los Angeles and, slightly further from home
base, 100 members of the World Presidents Organization (a diverse and successful international organization of
CEOs) meeting all the way up at the North Pole. The routine is safe and doable and includes segments that reduce
stress and increase strength, flexibility, and overall pep and
vitality.

Starting Off Slowly and Wisely

Most people find that they can successfully incorporate 15 to 20 minutes of practicing a new endeavor into their day on a regular basis. This chapter provides you with a short *asana* routine about that length designed to help you jump-start your Yoga practice. By practicing this routine three to six times per week, you'll notice improvements in your flexibility, muscle tone and strength, and concentration. Very likely, you'll notice a number of other benefits as well, such as better stamina, digestion, and sleep.

When practicing the postures that we describe in the following section, either follow the directions for breath and movement or simply stay in each posture for six to eight breaths.

 Because this may be your first Yoga experience — and you may have turned directly to this chapter — following is a quick trip through some basic Yoga principles you want to keep in mind:

- **Yoga isn't competitive.** Be patient. If you follow the directions, you will improve over time no matter what your starting level.

- **Move slowly into and out of the postures.** Never rush your Yoga session. Remember that coming out of a posture is an integral part of the posture itself.

- **Use yogic breathing throughout the routine and pause briefly after each inhalation and exhalation.** Chapter 5 gives you more info on yogic breathing.

- **Challenge but don't strain yourself.** Yoga should never hurt or cause you pain. Check out Chapters 2 and 3 for more on the proper Yoga attitude.

✔ **Move smoothly into and out of a posture several times before holding the posture.** Doing so prepares your body for a deeper stretch and helps you concentrate on linking the body, breath, and mind as we discuss in Chapter 5.

✔ **Don't change the order of the sequence and just randomly pick the postures you want.** All the routines have a special order or sequence to give you the maximum benefits. (For details about how to put together your own routines, see Chapter 15.)

Trying Out a Fun Beginner Routine

As you perform the postures in this short routine, notice how you start by giving your body and mind a chance to transition from your prior activity, how you move your body in several different directions, and how you end the routine with rest. These are some of the fundamental elements of a well-balanced Yoga routine, regardless of its length. Use focus breathing (which we cover in Chapter 5) throughout the routine.

Corpse posture

1. **Lie flat on your back with your arms relaxed along the sides of your torso and your palms up as shown in Figure 14-1.**

Figure 14-1:
Corpse
posture.

2. **Inhale and exhale through your nose slowly for 8 to 10 breaths.**

Pause briefly after each inhalation and exhalation.

Lying arm raise

1. **Lie in the corpse posture (see the preceding section) with your arms relaxed at your sides and your palms down as Figure 14-2a illustrates.**

Figure 14-2:
Lying arm raise.

2. **As you inhale, slowly raise your arms up overhead and touch the floor behind you as in Figure 14-2b.**

Pause briefly.

3. **As you exhale, bring your arms back to your sides as in Step 1.**

4. **Repeat Steps 2 and 3 six to eight times.**

Knee-to-chest posture

1. **Lie on your back with your knees bent and your feet flat on the floor.**

2. **As you exhale, bring your right knee into your chest and extend your left leg down.**

   Hold your shin just below your knee (see Figure 14-3). If you have knee problems, hold the back of your thigh instead.

3. **Stay in Step 2 for 6 to 8 breaths and then repeat on the left side.**

Figure 14-3:
Knee-to-chest
posture.

Downward-facing dog

1. **Beginning on your hands and knees, place your hands directly under your shoulders, with your palms spread on the floor and your knees directly under your hips.**

   Straighten your arms, but don't lock your elbows. Figure 14-4a shows you an example.

Figure 14-4:
Downward-facing dog.

2. **As you exhale, lift and straighten (but don't lock) your knees.**

   As your hips lift, bring your head down to a neutral position so that your ears are between your arms as Figure 14-4b illustrates. If possible, press your heels to the floor and your head toward your feet (stop if doing so strains your neck).

3. **As you inhale, come back down to your hands and knees as in Step 1.**

4. **Repeat Steps 1 through 3 three times and then stay in Step 2 for 6 to 8 breaths.**

Child's posture

1. **Starting on your hands and knees, place your knees about hip width apart with your hands just below your shoulders.**

   You want your elbows straight but not locked.

2. **As you exhale, sit back on your heels; rest your torso on your thighs and your forehead on the floor.**

   You don't have to sit all the way back.

3. Lay your arms back on the floor beside your torso with your palms up or reach your relaxed arms forward with your palms on the floor.

4. Close your eyes and stay in the folded position for 6 to 8 breaths (see Figure 14-5).

Figure 14-5:
Child's posture.

Warrior I

1. **Stand in the mountain posture (refer to Chapter 7) and step forward about 3 to 3 1/2 feet (or the length of one leg) with your right foot as you exhale.**

   Turn your left foot out (so the toes point to the left) if you need more stability.

2. **Place your hands on the top of your hips and square the front of your pelvis.**

   Release your hands and hang your arms as shown in Figure 14-6a.

3. **As you inhale, raise your arms forward and overhead and bend your right knee to a right angle so that it's directly over your ankle and your thigh is parallel to the floor.**

Check out Figure 14-6b for an illustration.

Figure 14-6:
Warrior I.

4. **Soften your arms (see Chapter 3 for a description of Forgiving Limbs) and face your palms toward each other.**

   If your lower back is uncomfortable, lean your torso slightly over the forward leg until your back releases any tension that may be present. Look straight ahead.

5. **Repeat Steps 3 and 4 three times and then hold once on the right side for 6 to 8 breaths.**

6. **Repeat Steps 1 through 5 on the other (left) side.**

Standing forward bend

1. **Start in the mountain posture (refer to Chapter 7) and raise your arms forward and then up overhead as you inhale (see Figure 14-7a).**

2. **As you exhale, bend forward from the hips.**

   When you feel a pull in the back of your legs, soften your knees (see Chapter 3 for information about

Forgiving Limbs) and hang your arms like in Figure 14-7b.

If your head isn't close to your knees, bend your knees more. If you have the flexibility, straighten your knees while keeping them soft. Relax your head and neck downward.

3. **Exhaling, roll your body up like a rag doll, stacking your vertebrae one at a time.**

Flip to Chapter 8 for more advanced ways to come up from a forward bend.

4. **Repeat Steps 1 through 3 three times and then stay down in Step 2 for 6 to 8 breaths.**

Figure 14-7:
Standing forward bend.

a   b

Reverse triangle posture

1. **Stand in the mountain posture (covered in Chapter 7) and step out to the right about 3 to 3 1/2 feet (or the length of one leg) with the right foot as you exhale.**

2. **As you inhale, raise your arms out to the sides**

parallel to the line of your shoulders (and the floor) so that your shoulders form a *T* with your torso as shown in Figure 14-8a.

3. **As you exhale, bend forward from the hips and then place your right hand on the floor near the inside of your left foot.**

Figure 14-8:
Reverse triangle posture.

4. **Raise your left arm toward the ceiling and look up at your left hand as Figure 14-8b illustrates.**

   Soften your knees and arms. Bend your left knee or move your right hand away from your left foot and more directly under your torso if you experience strain or discomfort.

5. **Repeat Steps 2 through 4 to the same side three times and then stay down in Step 4 for 6 to 8 breaths.**

6. **Repeat Steps 1 through 5 on the right side.**

You can strengthen or strain your neck in this posture, so turn your neck down if you're uncomfortable.

Standing spread-legged forward bend

1. Stand in the mountain posture (see Chapter 7) and step out to the right about 3 to 3 1/2 feet (or the length of one leg) with your right foot as you exhale.

2. As you inhale, raise your arms out to the sides parallel to the line of your shoulders (and the floor) so that your shoulders form a *T* with your torso as Figure 14-9a illustrates.

Figure 14-9:
Standing spread-legged forward bend.

3. As you exhale, bend forward from the hips and soften your knees.

4. Hold your bent elbows with the opposite-side hands and hang your torso and arms.

5. Stay folded in this posture (shown in Figure 14-9b) for 6 to 8 breaths.

The karate kid

1. Stand in the mountain posture (discussed in Chapter 7) and raise your arms out to the sides

287

parallel to the line of your shoulders (and the floor) so that your shoulders form a *T* with your torso as you inhale.

2. **Steady yourself and focus on a spot on the floor 10 to 12 feet in front of you.**

3. **As you exhale, bend and raise your left knee toward your chest, keeping your right leg straight as shown in Figure 14-10, and hold for 6 to 8 breaths.**

Figure 14-10:
The karate kid.

4. **Repeat Steps 1 through 3 with your legs reversed.**

After you become stable in the karate kid posture, try extending your bent left leg forward and up. Gradually work towards fully extending your left leg parallel to the floor — take your time! Try this added step on both sides.

Corpse posture redux

Repeat the corpse posture exercise as described in the earlier "Corpse posture" section and Figure 14-1. Stay for 8

288

to 12 breaths or choose one of the relaxation techniques in Chapter 4.

Reaching Beyond the Beginning

After you become comfortable with the beginners' routine in this chapter, you can expand it and add variety by following the guidelines we present in Chapter 15, where we walk you through designing your own Yoga program. If you're young and fit, you may want to try the routines in Chapter 17. If you're at mid life or older or haven't exercised for a while, Chapter 18 provides less strenuous (but equally beneficial) routines.

Of course, with a taste of Hatha Yoga, you may want to take private lessons or go to a group class for feedback, to boost your morale, or simply to practice — with new confidence — in the company of others.

Practicing on your own is fine, but nothing replaces working with a teacher. Before you get into too much of a Yoga groove, we recommend that you ask a Yoga teacher to check for any bad postural habits and, if you like, to give you some suggestions for taking the next step.

Part III
Creative Yoga

The 5th Wave   By Rich Tennant

YOGA SEQUENCE TO AVOID

WARM-UP

MAIN POSTURE

COMPENSATION POSTURE

REST

In this part . . .

Variety is the spice of life, and we trust you'll soon progress to the point of wanting to mix your beginners' routine up a little. In this part, we reveal the elements you need to design your own routines using postures you're already familiar with and more.

We also show you how Yoga suits people of all ages and stages — pregnancy, childhood, the young and restless, and the golden years, with some examples to help you and yours get started. We end with a no-nonsense discussion of props, which can be helpful aids in your practice.

Chapter 15

Designing Your Own Yoga Program

The art and science of sequencing in Yoga is called *vinyasa-krama* (pronounced *veen-yah-sah-krah-mah*). In the Sanskrit language, the word *vinyasa* means "placement" and *krama* means "step" or "process." This concept is often called "flow." The flow of postures is very important, and paying attention to proper sequencing can help you derive maximum benefit from your Hatha Yoga session.

Before you experiment with various Yoga postures, you need to know how to combine postures correctly. The more you know about sequencing, the better. Understanding sequencing is like figuring out how to unlock the door of a bank vault. You may have a list of all of the correct numbers, but if you don't know the correct combination, you can never open the door to the treasures hidden in the vault. In this chapter, we give you the secret combination, the essential rules for postural sequencing, so that you can create a Yoga program that's just right for you.

If you're dealing with a specific health challenge, you need to work one-on-one, under the guidance of your doctor, with a Yoga therapist or other health professional. This chapter focuses on "do-it-yourself" Hatha Yoga for general conditioning and stress reduction. Our emphasis is on prevention rather than therapy.

Applying the Rules of Sequencing

The sequence of postures depends on the overall format of your Yoga session, which in turn depends on your specific goals. What do you have in mind for your Yoga practice? What do you expect to accomplish? Are you interested in a simple stress reduction program, or do you want to put together a routine for general conditioning? After you establish your goal, you need a plan that can bring you safely and intelligently to your goal. A good plan includes these considerations:

- Your starting point
- Your next activity
- Your available time

Taking these factors into consideration helps you remain in the moment during your practice session.

After you establish your goals, you're ready to apply the rules of sequencing to achieve the best possible flow of exercises. Sequencing has many approaches, and we encourage you to consult a qualified teacher. (See Chapter 2 for more on setting goals and picking a teacher.) However, you can't go wrong when you bear in mind the following four basic categories:

- ✔ Warm-up or preparation
- ✔ Main postures
- ✔ Compensation
- ✔ Rest

Know thy schedule

Early in my teaching career, before I (Larry) had learned sequencing, I received a call from a high-level, highly stressed executive at a major corporation to arrange a private Yoga session in his office. I taught him a 30-minute routine and then asked him to lie on the floor with his feet up on a chair. I covered his eyes, recommended long exhalations, and then gave him a long, guided relaxation. He became so relaxed and looked so comfortable that I didn't want to disturb him when it was time for me to leave. He had already paid me, so I left thinking he'd appreciate continuing the relaxation on his own. What I didn't know was that he was giving a presentation shortly after the class. His secretary had to wake him in a hurry, and he was so spaced out for his presentation that he was even accused of being on drugs. The moral of the story: Never pay your Yoga instructor ahead of time. Just kidding. The true moral is that you should always take your next activity into account when designing your Yoga session.

Follow each step-by-step instruction carefully to avoid injuring yourself and also to enjoy maximum benefits. Always move into and out of the posture slowly, and pause after the inhalation and exhalation; we give you the details on correct breathing in Chapter 5.

The first part of this chapter includes some sample warm-up, compensation, and rest postures. The main postures are covered earlier in the book and are referred to throughout the chapter. The latter part of the chapter gives you a recipe to design your own Yoga routine using these concepts.

Getting Started with Warm-Ups

Any physical exercise requires adequate warm-up, and Yoga is no exception. Warm-up exercises increase circulation to the parts of your body that you're about to use and make you more aware of those areas of your physical self. What's different about the Yoga warm-up (called *preparation postures*) is that you do it slowly and deliberately with conscious breathing and awareness. It's integral to the Yoga session.

Here are some of the benefits of yogic warm-up:

- ✔ Brings awareness and presence of mind

- ✔ Allows you to test your body before executing the postures

- ✔ Increases the temperature and blood supply to your muscles, joints, and connective tissue

- ✔ Prepares your body for more challenging demands and reduces the possibility of muscle tear or strain

- ✔ Enhances the supply of oxygen and nutrients, thus

providing more stamina for the practice

✔ Prevents muscle soreness

You typically perform warm-up postures *dynamically,* which means you move in and out of them. In general, the safest Yoga warm-ups are simple forward bends and easy sequences that fold and unfold the body. Figure 15-1 shows some of our recommended warm-up exercises. You may select from the various reclining, sitting, and standing positions in this chapter. Normally, two or three postures are used for an adequate warm-up.

 If you have disc problems in your lower back, forward bends may not be a good way to warm-up. Check with your medical or chiropractic doctor.

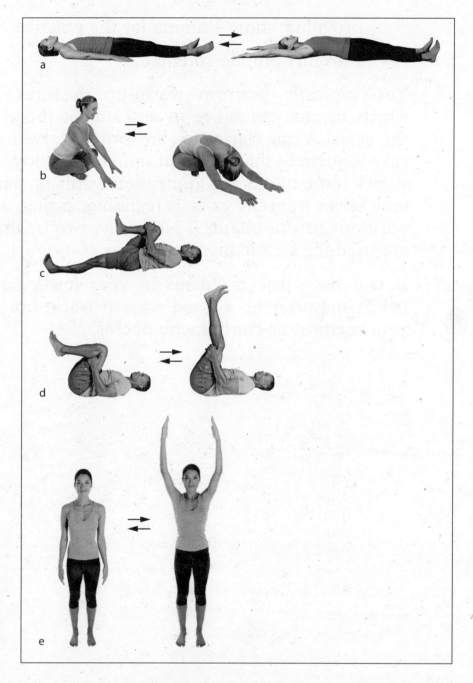

Figure 15-1:
Warm-up usually includes gentle bending and extending.

Warm-up or preparation postures are also used throughout a given routine to precede and enhance the effect of the main postures. (See Figure 15-2 for some samples.) For example, the leg lift just before a seated forward bend to stretch the hamstrings; the bridge posture just prior to a shoulder stand.

Avoid warming up with more complex postures such as shoulder stands (see Figure 15-3a), advanced back bends (Figure 15-3b), or deep twists (Figure 15-3c). Also, we suggest avoiding a heavy cardiovascular workout before a strenuous Yoga practice because you can experience muscle cramps.

Figure 15-3:
Avoid warming up with complex postures.

Reclining warm-up postures

Most Yoga practitioners enjoy reclining *(supine)* exercises because the postures are intrinsically relaxing. When you pair them with warm-ups, the combination effectively allows you to warm-up specific muscles or muscle groups while keeping the other muscles at rest. You're having your cake and eating it too.

The following warm-up exercises require you to start with the corpse posture (or dead posture), which we describe in Chapter 4. These exercises help revive you even when you start your Yoga session dead tired (pun intended).

Lying arm raise

Many of the muscles that go to the neck start between your shoulder blades. Raising the arms brings circulation to frequent sites of tension. You can see an illustration in Figure 15-1a.

1. **Lie flat on your back with your arms relaxed at your sides and your palms turned down.**

2. **As you inhale, slowly raise your arms over your**

head and touch the floor.

3. As you exhale, bring your arms back to your sides as in Step 1.

4. Repeat Steps 1 through 3, six to eight times.

The double breath

If you want to double your pleasure, the double breath enhances tension release in your body and prepares your muscles for the main postures.

1. Repeat Steps 1 and 2 of the lying arm raise in the preceding section.

2. After you raise your arms overhead on the inhalation, leave them on the floor above your head and fully exhale.

   Your arms should remain where they are for another inhalation while you deeply stretch your entire body from the tips of your toes to your fingertips.

3. On the next exhalation, return your arms to your sides and relax your legs; repeat 3 to 4 times.

Knee-to-chest posture

Use this exercise for either warm-up or compensation. The knee-to-chest posture is also a classic in lower-back programs (see Chapter 22 for more on Yoga therapy for low-back troubles). Figure 15-1c shows you what it looks like.

1. Lie on your back with your knees bent and feet flat on the floor.

2. As you exhale, bring your right knee into your

chest, holding your shin just below your knee.

If you have knee problems, hold the back of your thigh rather than your shin.

3. **If you can do so comfortably, straighten your left leg on the floor.**

   If you have back problems, though, keep your left knee bent.

4. **Repeat Steps 1 through 3 on the other side, holding each side for 6 to 8 breaths.**

Double leg extension

This exercise, which uses both legs simultaneously, has a dual function. It prepares the lower back and gently stretches the hamstrings.

Check it out in Figure 15-1c.

1. **Lie on your back and bring your bent knees toward your chest.**

2. **Hold the backs of your thighs at arms' length.**

3. **As you inhale, straighten both legs perpendicular to the floor; as you exhale, bend both legs again.**

4. **Repeat Steps 2 and 3 six to eight times.**

Hamstring stretch

Without the hamstrings (the muscles and the associated tendons), you'd have to let your fingers do all the walking. The hamstrings can be injured quite easily, especially if you overwork them, so you want to prepare them properly for exercise. Refer to Figure 15-4 for a visual.

1. **Lying on your back with your legs straight, place your arms along your sides with your palms down.**

2. **Bend just your left knee and put that foot on the floor (see Figure 15-4a).**

3. **As you exhale, bring your right leg up as straight as possible (see Figure 15-4b). As you inhale, return your right leg to the floor.**

   Keep your head and your hips on the floor.

4. **Repeat Steps 3 and 4 three times and then, with your hands interlocked on the back of your raised thigh just above your knee, hold your leg in place for 6 to 8 breaths (see Figure 15-4c).**

5. **Repeat Steps 1 through 4 on the other side.**

Figure 15-4:
Unlock your hamstrings, and you open the door to many Yoga postures.

Support your head with a pillow or folded blanket if the back of your neck or your throat tenses when you raise or lower your leg.

Dynamic bridge: Dvipada pitha

You can use this exercise for warm-up and compensation and as a main posture. The Sanskrit term *dvipada* means "two-footed" and *pitha* means "seat," which is a synonym for *asana.* (The pronunciation is *dvee-pah-dah peet-hah.*)

1. **Lie on your back with your knees bent, feet flat on the floor at hip width, and your arms at your sides with palms turned down (see Figure 15-5a).**

2. **As you inhale, raise your hips to a comfortable height (see Figure 15-5b).**

3. **As you exhale, return your hips to the floor.**

4. **Repeat Steps 3 and 4 six to eight times.**

Figure 15-5: *The dynamic bridge.*

Bridge variation with arm raise

This posture is another good candidate for both warm-up and compensation.

1. **Lie on your back with your knees bent, your feet flat on the floor at hip width, and your arms at your sides with palms turned down (refer to Figure 15-5a).**

2. As you inhale, raise your hips to a comfortable height and at the same time raise your arms overhead to touch the floor (see Figure 15-6).

3. As you exhale, return your hips to the floor and your arms to your sides.

4. Repeat Steps 3 and 4 six to eight times.

Figure 15-6: Bridge variation with arm raise.

Dynamic head-to-knee

The dynamic head-to-knee is a nice warm-up before a slightly more physical routine.

Dynamic head-to-knee is a little more vigorous kind of warm-up. Don't perform this sequence if you're having neck problems.

1. Lie flat on your back with your arms relaxed at your sides and you palms turned down as shown in Figure 15-1a earlier in the chapter.

2. As you inhale, raise your arms slowly overhead and touch the floor.

3. As you exhale, draw your right knee toward your chest, lift your head off the floor, and then grasp your right knee with your hands.

   Keep your hips on the floor. Bring your head as

close to your knee as possible, but don't force it. Figure 15-7 shows you what this position looks like.

4. **As you inhale, release your knee and return your head, arms, and straightened right leg to the floor as they are in Step 2.**

5. **Repeat Steps 2 through 4 six to eight times on each side, alternating right and left.**

To make the sequence a little easier, keep your head on the floor in Step 3.

Figure 15-7:
The dynamic head-to-knee.

Standing warm-up postures

The standing postures are probably the most versatile of all the groups. They can be used for warm-up/preparation, compensation, or as main postures. As a warm-up, use standing postures when the next part of your routine is also performed from a standing position.

Standing arm raise

You can perform this versatile warm-up (shown in Figure 15-1e) almost anywhere you want to enjoy a complete break from sitting. Try it at the office and start a new trend.

1. **Stand tall but relaxed with your feet at hip width.**

2. **Hang your arms at your sides with your palms turned back.**

   Look straight ahead.

3. **As you inhale, raise your arms forward and then up overhead.**

4. **As you exhale, bring your arms down and back to your sides.**

5. **Repeat Steps 3 and 4 six to eight times.**

The head-turner

Sequences like the head-turner combine breath and movement in parts of the upper body to stretch, strengthen, and heal your entire wingspan. This breath and movement sequence for the upper back and neck is great for minor stiff necks.

1. **Stand tall but relaxed with your feet at hip width.**

2. **Hang your arms at your sides, palms turned back.**

   Look straight ahead.

3. **As you inhale, raise your right arm forward and up overhead as you turn your head to the left as Figure 15-8 illustrates.**

4. **As you exhale, bring your arm down and turn your head forward.**

5. **As you inhale, raise your left arm forward and**

up overhead while turning your head to the right.

6. **Repeat Steps 3 through 5 six to eight times on each side, alternating right and left.**

Figure 15-8:
The
head-turner.

Shoulder rolls

Shoulder rolls are used in many types of exercise routines; but when done in Yoga, you move slowly and with awareness, coordinating with the breath.

1. **Stand tall but relaxed with your feet at hip width.**

2. **Hang your arms at your sides with your palms turned back.**

   Look straight ahead.

3. **As you inhale, roll your shoulders up and back**

as shown in Figure 15-9. As you exhale, drop your shoulders down.

4. Repeat Step 3 six to eight times, reversing the direction of the rolls.

Figure 15-9:
Move slowly in the shoulder rolls, coordinating breath and movement.

Dynamic standing forward bend

Like many other warm-ups, you can also use this exercise for compensation.

1. Stand tall but relaxed with your feet at hip width.

2. Hang your arms at your sides with your palms turned back.

3. As you inhale, raise your arms forward and up overhead (see Figure 15-10a).

4. As you exhale, bend forward, and when you feel

a pull in the back of your legs, bend your legs and arms slightly (see Figure 15-10b).

This position is called Forgiving Limbs, and we cover it in Chapter 3.

5. **As you inhale, roll up slowly, stacking the bones of your spine one at a time from bottom to top; then raise your arms overhead and finally, release your arms back to your sides.**

6. **Repeat Steps 3 through 5 six to eight times.**

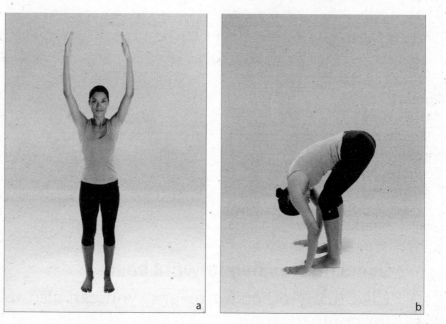

Figure 15-10:
Feel free to soften your knees in the dynamic standing forward bend.

 Rolling up is the safest way to come up in Step 5. If you don't have back problems, you may want to try two more advanced techniques after a few weeks: As you come up, sweep your arms out and up from the sides like wings, then overhead. Alternately, as you inhale, extend your slightly bent arms forward and up until they're parallel with your ears. Then raise your upper back, your mid back, and then your lower back until you're all the way up and your arms are overhead.

Seated warm-up postures

Yoga postures provide a very broad spectrum of possibilities. You can do an entire routine from a seated position, including forward bends, back bends, side bends, and twists. In this section, we show you how to prepare for main postures from a seated position. (**Note:** Most of the postures here utilize the easy posture, *sukhasana*. Check out that discussion in Chapter 6.)

Seated fold

The seated fold is a very simple way to warm-up your back for forward bends or to compensate after seated twists.

1. **Sit on the floor with your legs crossed in the easy posture and place your hands on the floor in front of you with palms down (refer to Figure 15-1b for a visual).**

2. **As you exhale, slide your hands out along the floor and bend forward at the hips.**

   If possible, bring your head down to the floor; otherwise, just come as close as you comfortably can.

3. **As you inhale, roll your torso and head up and return to the starting position in Step 1.**

4. **Repeat Steps 2 and 3 four to six times and then switch your legs and repeat four to six times.**

If you have a disc-related back problem, exercise caution with forward bends.

Rock the baby

This series prepares you for advanced sitting postures and forward bends.

1. **Sit on the floor with your legs stretched out in front of you.**

   Press your hands on the floor behind you for support

2. **Shake your legs out.**

3. **Bend your right knee and place your right foot just above your left knee with your right ankle to the outside of the left knee (see Figure 15-11a).**

4. **Stabilize your right foot with your left hand and your right knee with your right hand; swing your right knee up and down 6 to 8 times by gently pressing and then releasing the inner right thigh.**

5. **Carefully lift your right foot up and cradle it in the crook of your left elbow; cradle your right knee in the crook of your right elbow and, if you can, interlock your fingers (see Figure 15-11b).**

6. **Lift your spine and rock your right leg gently side to side 6 to 8 times.**

7. **Repeat Steps 1 through 6 with the left leg.**

8. **Shake your legs out.**

If you can't do this sequence without pain, don't try the more advanced seated postures in Chapter 6. Moreover, we don't recommend the rock the baby sequence if you have knee or hip problems.

Figure 15-11:
Rock the baby.

a

b

Selecting Your Main Postures and Compensation Poses

After your body is warmed up, you can move into what we refer to as the *main postures,* the central part of the routine. Interspersed between the main postures are *compensation postures,* which allow your body to come back into balance after each main posture and prevent discomfort and injury.

Getting stronger with standard asanas

The main postures are the standard *asanas* you find featured in the classical Yoga texts and modern manuals. These *asanas* are the stars of your routine, requiring you to work a little harder. The chapters of Part II describe many of the main postures that we recommend for beginners. Figure 15-12 shows you some examples. Whichever *asanas* you select, remember to match them with your specific goals.

Whenever possible, a warm-up posture precedes and a compensation posture follows each category of main postures.

The number of postures you select for your Yoga session depends on your available time and your goals. Later in this chapter, we provide you with a framework for selecting postures for varying lengths of time, as well as guidelines to create routines that focus on general conditioning, stress reduction, preparation for meditation, and a quick pick-me-up.

then

then

then

then

then

then

Figure 15-12:
Compensation postures.

315

Bringing balance with compensation postures

Compensation is part of bringing you back into balance, which is a key concept in Yoga. Use compensation postures to unwind or bring your body back into neutral, especially after strenuous postures.

Here are some basic guidelines for using compensation postures:

- Use one or two simple compensation postures to neutralize tension you feel in any area of the body after a Yoga posture or sequence.

- Always use the conscious breathing we describe in Chapter 5.

- Perform compensating postures that are simpler or less difficult than the main posture right after the main posture. Do them dynamically.

- Don't follow a strenuous posture with another strenuous posture in the opposite direction. Some Yoga instructors teach the fish posture as compensating for the shoulder stand. However, this combination can cause problems, especially for beginners, so we recommend the less strenuous cobra posture instead.

- Use compensation postures even when you feel no immediate need for them, especially after deep back bends, twists, and inverted postures.

- Gentle forward bends typically compensate back bends, twists, and side bends.

- Many forward bends are self-compensating. However, we follow with gentle back bends after doing a lot of forward bending.

✔ Rest after strenuous postures, such as inverted postures or deep back bends, before beginning the compensation postures.

Following are some great compensation postures.

The dynamic cat

The dynamic cat is a very nice compensation posture for twists, but you can also use it for warm-up.

1. **Starting on your hands and knees, look straight ahead.**

2. **Place your knees at hip width with your hands below your shoulders (see Figure 15-13a).**

    Straighten but don't lock your elbows.

3. **As you exhale, sit back on your heels and look at the floor (see Figure 15-13b).**

4. **As you inhale, slowly return to the starting position in Step 1.**

    Again, look straight ahead.

5. **Repeat Steps 3 and 4 six to eight times.**

Figure 15-13:
Dynamic cat.

Dynamic knees-to-chest

You can find many variations of knees-to-chest (including the regular version later in this chapter), but this variation is especially good after back bends.

1. **Lie on your back and bend your knees toward your chest.**

2. **Hold your legs just below your knees, one hand on each leg (see Figure 15-14a).**

   If you have any knee problems, be sure to hold the backs of your thighs.

3. **As you exhale, draw your knees toward your chest (see Figure 15-14b).**

4. **As you inhale, move your knees away from your chest.**

5. **Repeat Steps 3 and 4 six to eight times.**

Figure 15-14:
Dynamic knees-to-chest.

Thunderbolt posture: Vajrasana

This exercise is useful for compensation or warm-up. *Vajra* (pronounced *vahj-rah*) means both "diamond/adamantine" and "thunderbolt."

1. **Kneel on the floor with your knees and feet at hip width.**

2. **Sit back on your heels and bring your back up nice and tall. Hang your arms close to your sides.**

3. **As you inhale, lift your hips back up and sweep your arms up over your head (see Figure 15-15a).**

   Lean back and look up.

4. **As you exhale, sit on your heels again, fold your chest to your thighs, and bring your arms behind your back (see Figure 15-15b).**

   Get into a nice flow. Inhale when you open, exhale when you fold.

5. **Repeat Steps 3 and 4 six to eight times.**

Don't perform the thunderbolt if you have knee problems.

Figure 15-15:
The thunderbolt posture.

Including Plenty of Rest and Relaxation

Rest periods are an indispensable part of any good Yoga routine. Rest isn't just zoning out at the end of a session. In Yoga, a quiet interval is an active tool for enhancing the quality of your practice at the following times:

- ✔ Before the beginning of a class to shift gears and establish a union between your body, breath, and mind

- ✔ Between postures to renew and prepare for the next posture

- ✔ As part of compensation after strenuous postures

- ✔ To restore proper breathing

- ✔ For self-observation

- ✔ To prepare for relaxation techniques

Knowing when to rest and when to resume

 The two best indicators of the need to rest are your *breath* and *energy level*. Monitor yourself throughout the session. If your breath is loud and uneven, rest. If you feel a little tired after a posture, rest.

No formula can prescribe how long you need to rest. Simply rest as needed until you're ready for the next posture. Don't cheat yourself out of well-deserved rest periods between the postures and at the end of a session.

Rest postures

Figure 15-16 shows you some recommended rest postures.

Stay in any rest posture for 6 to 12 breaths or as long as it takes to feel rested, which may depend on how much time you have and where you are in the sequence of the routine. Yoga should never feel like you're in a hurry.

Corpse posture: Shavasana

The word *shava* (pronounced *shah-vah*) means "corpse"; this posture is also called the dead pose or *mritasana*, from *mrita* (pronounced *mree-tah*) meaning "dead" and *asana* meaning "posture." Refer to Figure 15-16a and Chapter 4 for a full description of the posture.

Figure 15-16:
You can rest in many different positions.

Shavasana variation with bent legs

Follow the steps for *shavasana* in Chapter 4 but keep your knees bent with your feet on the floor at hip width as shown in Figure 15-16b.

 If your back is uncomfortable, place a pillow or blanket roll under your knees. If your neck or throat is tense, place a folded blanket or small pillow under your head.

Easy posture: Sukhasana

The word *sukha* means "easy" or "pleasant" and indeed this posture is as its name suggests. You can keep your eyes open or closed in this posture. Check out Figure 15-16c and Chapter 6 for more details.

Mountain posture: Tadasana

The Sanskrit word *tada* (pronounced *tah-dah*) actually means "palm tree"; hence, this exercise is also called the palm tree posture.

1. **Stand tall but relaxed with your feet at hip width.**

   Your arms are at your sides with your palms turned toward the sides of the legs.

2. **Visualize a vertical line connecting the hole in your ear, your shoulder joint, and the sides of your hip, knee, and ankle.**

3. **Look straight ahead with your eyes open or closed, as Figure 15-16d illustrates.**

Child's posture: Balasana

The Sanskrit word *bala* (pronounced *bah-lah*) means

"child." This classic version of child's posture is a very nurturing pose.

1. **Start on your hands and knees.**

2. **Place your knees about hip width, hands just below your shoulders.**

   Keep your elbows straight but not locked.

3. **As you exhale, sit back on your heels; rest your torso on your thighs and your forehead on the floor.**

4. **Lay your arms on the floor beside your torso with your palms up as shown in Figure 15-16e.**

5. **Close your eyes and breathe easily.**

Child's posture with arms in front

This variation of child's posture gives you more stretch in your upper back. Follow the steps for the child's posture in the preceding section but extend your arms forward at Step 4, spreading your palms on the floor as Figure 15-16f illustrates.

Knees-to-chest posture: Apanasana

The Sanskrit word *apana* (pronounced *ah-pah-nah*) refers to the downward-going life force or exhalation.

1. **Lie on your back and bend your knees in toward your chest.**

2. **Hold your shins just below the knees as in Figure 15-16g.**

   If you have any knee problems, hold the backs of your thighs instead.

Cooking Up a Creative Yoga Routine with the Classic Formula

When you create your own Yoga program with our classic formula, you

✔ Determine how long you want the routine to be

✔ Select the main postures from the range of postures covered in Chapters 6 through 13 (or, of course, from any source you consider reliable)

✔ Decide how you want to prepare and/or compensate for each main category of postures

✔ Allocate time for rest and for relaxation at the end in order to digest the nutritious meal of Yoga exercises that you prepared for yourself

 What we call the Classic Formula consists of the following 12 categories:

1. Attunement (integrating body, breath, and mind)

2. Warm-up/preparation (also used between main exercises wherever necessary)

3. Standing postures

4. Balance postures (optional)

5. Abdominals

6. Inversions (optional)

7. Back bends

8. Forward bends

9. Twists

10. Rest (to be inserted between main exercises whenever you feel the need)

11. Compensation (to be inserted after main exercises)

12. Final relaxation

You don't have to use every category as long as you follow the proper sequence from 1 to 9 and always conclude with 12. Depending on your available time, you may choose to omit number 4 or 6 and continue, or even stop the asanas after number 5 if time is short and jump to step 12. You can repeat the categories of rest, warm-up/preparation, and compensation wherever appropriate. Balancing postures and inversions are optional because their inclusion depends on your available time, wallspace, and your skill level.

The Classic Formula is optimal for 30- to 60-minute general conditioning programs, but we also refer to it in the 15- and 5-minute programs. The beauty of our formula is that as your Yoga practice grows over the years, you can explore safe postures from any book or system and then insert them into their appropriate slots within our 12-category module.

A postural feast: The 30- to 60-minute general-conditioning routine

Most beginning Yoga students find sustaining more than a 30-minute practice on their own difficult; however, if your appetite increases, we want you to have the tools to be a 60-minute gourmet. Simply follow the recipes in each of the categories to create your own great, custom routine.

 Plan for an average of about two minutes for each posture you select. Some postures take more time, some take less. Doing both sides of an *asymmetrical* or one-side-at-a-time (right and left) posture like the warrior (see Chapter 7) is counted as one exercise or posture. If you choose our sun salutation or a similar dynamic series from Chapters 13 and 15 or another source, double or triple the time allotted depending on the series and the number of repetitions.

Note: As we indicate throughout this chapter, you can use many of these postures in more than one category when developing a general-conditioning routine.

 The simplest way to expand a 30-minute routine into a 45-minute routine is to do two sets of your chosen standing postures and add one extra posture to the abdominal, back bend, and forward bend categories.

Attunement

Attunement allows you to establish the conscious link between your body, breath, and mind or awareness. If you forget about the attunement stage, you miss much of what makes Yoga, Yoga.

First, for routines of any length, select a style of breathing from Chapter 5. If you're a beginner, choose something simple like focus breathing or belly breathing. Later you can try either the classic three-part breathing or chest-to-belly breathing or adopt the *ujjayi* technique.

 Be sure not to confuse these styles of breathing with the traditional techniques of breath control *(pranayama)* that we also describe in Chapter 5.

Next, select one of the resting postures from earlier in this chapter or a seated posture from Chapter 6, depending on your frame of mind, physical condition, or what you have planned for the rest of your routine. The corpse posture (lying flat on your back) is always a good starting point for beginners. It's a great way to shift gears from a hectic lifestyle and slow things down before beginning your postural exercises. Lying flat on your back definitely shifts your mood toward relaxation. However, sitting in the easy posture or standing in the mountain posture are also great starting points. Figure 15-16 shows some examples of rest postures that you can use to help achieve attunement.

Use 8 to 12 breaths to achieve attunement. The more you pay attention to your breath and attunement, the more benefit you can expect to derive from your program. Think of the benefits you receive as "mileage plus."

Warm-up

You may notice that almost all the warm-ups we describe earlier in this chapter are folding and opening motions (flexion and extension). Either motion provides the easiest way for your body to prepare for breath and movement. Select a warm-up posture or sequence that is a similar position to your attunement posture.

 Make your Yoga practice as smooth as possible. Flow like a gentle river. For example, do both the attunement and warm-up on the floor; then stand for the next series of postures. Avoid getting up and down like a yo-yo. Economy of movement is one of the principles of good Hatha Yoga practice.

 In a routine of 30 minutes or more, you usually have time for at least two warm-up postures. Because the neck is a frequent site of tension, we suggest using a warm-up posture that incorporates moving the arms. In addition to stretching the spine, arm movement prepares your neck and shoulders and helps you release tension. Also, warm-ups that move the legs and prepare the lower back are helpful for the standing postures that usually follow. Check out "Getting Started with Warm-ups" earlier in the chapter for some examples of common warm-ups in the lying, sitting, and standing positions.

Standing postures

The standing postures tend to be the most physical part of a program. If you're doing a 30-minute routine, you usually have time for three or four standing postures. In a 60-minute program, you may have as many as six or seven standing *asanas*. You can choose any of the standing postures from Chapter 7 for this portion of your routine.

As a general rule back bends, twists, and side bends (the hallmarks of many standing postures) come before forward bends. Therefore, you want to include standing forward bends after most of the standing postures you choose.

Figure 15-17 shows you examples of standing postures for a 30- or 60-minute program. As an alternative, you can choose the dynamic kneeling or standing sequence (sun salutation) or the standing rejuvenation sequence for beginners from Chapter 13. The dynamic postures take the place of three to six standing postures, depending on which sequence you choose and how many rounds you do. When you select a dynamic sequence, try to allow time at the end for one twist and one compensating forward bend. We mention this note because all our dynamic sequences are forward and backward bends only.

If you want your routine to be more physically challenging, simply do two sets of the standing postures.

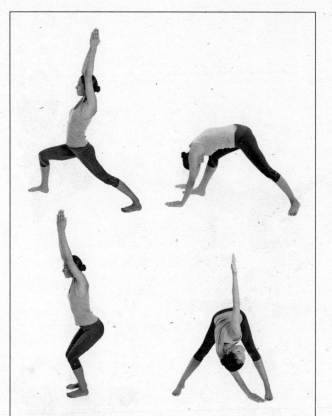

Figure 15-17:
Examples of popular standing postures.

Balancing postures (optional)

Balancing postures are optional and depend on your time and stamina. They're often the most athletic postures and require overall coordination. Balancing postures are very rewarding because you can see your progress immediately. They fit nicely after the standing postures because at this point in your routine, you're fully warmed up. All our recommended balancing postures are either standing or kneeling, which means they fit smoothly into the sequence. Choose one balancing posture from Chapter 8 for a 30-minute to 60-minute routine; Figure 15-18 shows you some options.

Figure 15-18:
You can practice balance from many different positions.

Rest

Most people usually welcome a rest at this point of the routine. Resting is usually done lying, sitting, or kneeling. We emphasize the importance of not feeling rushed during your Yoga session. At least for the short duration of your routine, believe that you have all the time in the world. In a 30- or 60-minute routine, the first rest usually comes at the halfway point. This resting period gives you the opportunity for inward observation of any physical, mental, or emotional feedback resulting from your Yoga practice so far.

Remember that you need to rest until you feel ready to move on. If you're really pinched for time, this first major rest is also a logical place to end a session. Choose from any of our recommended resting postures in Figure 15-16, or any of the sitting postures that you're comfortable with from Chapter 6.

Abdominals

We recommend that you include at least one (but not more than two) abdominal postures in any program lasting 30 minutes or more. Think of your abdomen as the front of your back — a very important place. Choose one of the abdominal postures we describe in Chapter 9 for a 30-minute routine or one or two for a 60-minute routine. You can check out some examples in Figure 15-19.

Figure 15-19: Practice your yogi ab postures with a slow, coordinated breath.

Compensation and preparation

Take a short rest when you finish the abdominal exercises and then do six to eight repetitions of the dynamic bridge or bridge variation (both discussed earlier in the chapter and shown in Figure 15-5) or the lying arm raise (also covered earlier). The action of the dynamic bridge plays a dual function here because it compensates the abdomen, returning it to neutral, and also warms up or prepares the back and the neck if you choose to include an inversion posture or move on to back bends next.

Inversion (optional)

Indian Yoga teachers often teach inverted postures toward the beginning or at the end of a class. For Westerners, we prefer to introduce inverted postures closer to the middle of the routine, when they've properly prepared their backs and necks and have plenty of time for adequate compensation. Inverted postures like those shown in Figure 15-20 are optional, and we recommend that beginners avoid the half shoulder stand and the half shoulder stand at the wall until they've practiced Yoga for six to eight weeks.

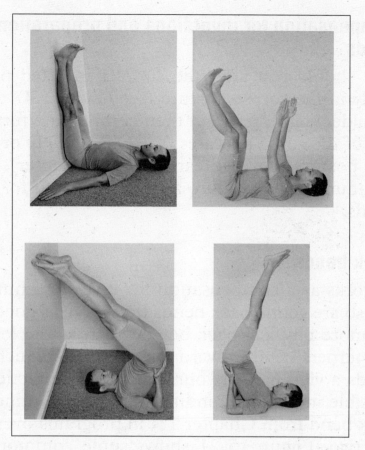

Figure 15-20:
Inversions are powerful postures that deserve respect.

Attempt inversions only if you have no neck problems. Inverted postures are worthy of a healthy respect. They're powerful postures that demand a sense of balance and strong muscles. We offer you several easy and safe inversion postures in Chapter 10. Select just one for your 30- to 60-minute routine, assuming you're ready and want to include an inversion in your practice.

Even if you are ready for an inversion, we advise against practicing the shoulder stand or the half shoulder stand at the wall if any of the following conditions applies to you: glaucoma, retinopathy, high blood pressure, a history of heart attacks or stroke, hiatal hernia, the first few days of menstruation, pregnancy, or 40 or more pounds of excess weight.

Compensation for inversions and preparation for back bends

You should rest after the simpler inverted postures, normally in the corpse posture (see Chapter 4). After the half shoulder stand, rest and then compensate further with any one of the cobra postures (see Chapter 11) or the thunderbolt posture (covered earlier in the chapter). Cobra I and the thunderbolt posture also prepare you for further back bends.

Back bends

It works as a compensation for inversion, but cobra I and II also are gentle back bends that serve as good preparation for more physical back bends, such as the locust posture. Westerners bend forward far too much, which makes back bends a vital part of your Hatha Yoga practice. Whenever possible in general-conditioning Yoga routines, select one back bend from Chapter 11; in programs over 30 minutes, use two. Figure 15-21 shows some common back bends you can try.

Figure 15-21:
Examples of four common back bends.

Compensation for back bends

The compensation for *prone* (lying face down) back bends is usually some form of a bent-knee forward bend (shown in Figure 15-22). We often recommend the knees-to-chest posture or the child's posture discussed earlier in the chapter. After more strenuous back bends, such as any of the varieties of the locust postures, we suggest a short rest followed by one of the bent-knee forward bends and then the dynamic bridge posture as a second compensatory posture. This sequence helps neutralize the upper back and neck.

Preparation for forward bends

Preparation is particularly critical for extended leg forward bends. Stretching the hamstrings or the hips just before doing a seated forward bend (refer to Chapter 11) not only improves the posture but is also safer for your back. Use the hamstring stretch or the double leg stretch for a 30-minute routine. (see Figure 15-4). For a longer routine, use both and/or the rock the baby sequence (see Figure 15-11).

Forward bends

The seated forward bends normally come toward the end of an exercise program because they have a calming effect. Of all the postures described in this book, the seated extended-leg forward bends divide the sexes the most. Because of their higher muscle density, especially in the hip and groin area, men are usually tighter in the hamstrings. Preparation of the hamstrings is particularly important for them in these postures. If you have a hard time with this category, bend your knees more and, if necessary, place some blankets under your hips to give yourself a better angle for the forward bends (which we cover in Chapter 11). For a 30-minute routine, choose just one forward bend from Chapter 11; pick two for a 60-minute routine. Figure 15-23 shows you some possibilities. Alternately, you may substitute with one kneeling or seated side bend from

Chapter 11, and one seated or kneeling forward bend from earlier in this chapter for compensation.

Compensation for forward bends

The forward bends are usually self-compensating. However, sometimes you may want to use a gentle back bend like the dynamic bridge as a counter pose.

Preparation for twists

The preparation for all twists is a forward bend, so moving from forward bends to twists flows naturally. Check out the earlier section "Forward bends" for guidance on choosing a bend.

Twists

Twists, like forward bends, have an overall calming effect; the floor twists are the dessert in our program, because at the end of the routine they feel so good. Choose one floor twist from Chapter 12 for a 30-minute routine and one or two for a 60-minute routine. Figure 15-24 shows some common twists.

Compensation for twists

Compensation for twists is always flexion, or a forward bend. After a floor twist, we usually recommend choosing one of the lying knees-to-chest or the regular knees-to-chest postures in Figure 15-13 and Figure 15-4 earlier in the chapter.

Relaxation

No matter how short your program, remember to include some form of relaxation. Rest provides a place where you digest all the marvelous energy unleashed by your Yoga exercises. It's like receiving "mileage plus" from your Yoga practice.

Figure 15-24:
Twists are calming postures, and they just plain feel good.

This final category in our classic formula can take several forms: a relaxation technique (see Chapter 4), *pranayama* yogic breathing (see Chapter 5), or meditation (see Chapter 21).

First, choose a rest posture or one of the seated postures from Chapter 6. Next, select one of the breathing or *pranayama* techniques from Chapter 5, a relaxation technique from Chapter 4, and/or a meditation technique from Chapter 21. In a 60-minute routine, you may choose both a breathing and a relaxation technique. Whichever technique you choose, use it for at least 2 to 3 minutes and not more than 15 minutes.

Making the most of a little: A 15-minute routine

Sometimes you have only 15 minutes, but even 15 minutes of Hatha Yoga can put you back on an even keel and refresh you.

When you opt for a 15-minute program, you need to be specific about your goals. Some of the more common uses for a short routine are

✔ A quick general-conditioning program

✔ A stress-reduction and relaxation program

✔ A preparation program for Yoga breathing or meditation.

General conditioning

For the purposes of general conditioning, choose the following categories and do them in the order listed. You can also use the illustrations earlier in this chapter as a reference point.

Some of the postures below appear in this chapter; you can also find information in the listed chapters.

- ✔ Either a standing or seated rest posture for attunement (flip to "Rest postures" earlier in this chapter as well as Chapters 6 and 7) and a Yoga breathing technique from Chapter 5.

- ✔ A dynamic series, such as either kneeling or standing sun salutation (Chapter 13); the rejuvenation sequence, which counts as three or four postures (also in Chapter 13) or three to four standing postures (see "Standing postures" earlier in this chapter plus Chapter 7) for six to eight minutes.

- ✔ A lying twist (see "Twists" earlier in this chapter as well as Chapter 12).

- ✔ Compensate with knees- or knee-to-chest postures (check out Figure 15-13 earlier in the chapter).

- ✔ A lying or seated rest posture from the "Rest postures" section earlier in the chapter.

- ✔ A breathing exercise from Chapter 5 and/or a relaxation technique from Chapter 4.

Preparation for meditation and Yoga breathing

If you're looking for a routine to help you reduce stress, just plain relax, or prepare for meditation and Yoga breathing, choose the following elements in the order listed:

- ✔ A lying or seated posture from this chapter's "Rest postures" section or Chapter 6 or 7 for attunement and a Yoga breathing technique from Chapter 5. Repeat this or a similar posture at the end of the routine.

- ✔ Two lying warm-up postures from "Getting Started with Warm-ups" earlier in the chapter — one that moves the arms and the other that moves the legs.

- ✔ A prone back-bending posture such as cobra I or locust I (see this chapter's "Back bends" and Chapter 11) or a lying back bend such as the bridge.

- ✔ A bent knee compensation exercise such as the child's posture or knees-to-chest posture covered in "Compensation for back bends" earlier in the chapter.

- ✔ A lying hamstring posture such as rock the baby, covered earlier in the chapter.

- ✔ A lying twist (see this chapter's "Twists" section as well as Chapter 12).

- ✔ A lying bent-knee compensation exercise as shown in Figure 15-14 earlier in the chapter.

Satisfy an appetite for a quick pick-me-up: A 5-minute routine

A 5-minute program is the easiest to create. For a busy person, even three to five minutes once or twice a day can provide beneficial effects. Settle into a rest posture or a seated posture from this chapter's "Rest postures" section or Chapter 6 and then employ a yogic breathing or *pranayama* technique (see Chapter 5) for three to five minutes. You can come up with many possible combinations for a quick, relaxing, and enjoyable routine.

Chapter 16

It's Never Too Soon: Pre- and Postnatal Yoga

In This Chapter

▶ Understanding Yoga's pregnancy benefits
▶ Exploring some good pregnancy postures (plus a routine)
▶ Easing back into Yoga postpartum

The value of regular exercise isn't lost just because you're pregnant. In fact, the American College of Obstetrics and Gynecology (ACOG) recommends that pregnant women become physically active to help alleviate some of the common discomforts associated with pregnancy, prepare for childbirth, and get back into shape afterward.

In this chapter, we discuss the benefits of Yoga practice during pregnancy, go through the best poses for a pregnant body, and provide a quick and easy routine to try.

Partnering Yoga with Pregnancy

Taking a gentle approach to Yoga during pregnancy can be

just what the doctor ordered. It may be just what the mid-wife ordered as well because it helps you cultivate a sense of confidence in your own body and your ability to give birth. Of course, each woman should consult her physician about her own needs just to be certain she doesn't have any high-risk conditions that may require special precautions.

We think that the best way to take full advantage of Yoga is to start your practice well before you're pregnant, or at least as soon as you receive the good news. Your Yoga practice can build a strong, healthy body and a stable mind, not only helping you conceive a child (by making you fit and relaxed) but also supporting you during the pregnancy, at birth, and afterwards. Many of our students continue their Yoga practice during their entire pregnancies, using the conservative principles that we outline in this book.

Womb with a (yogic) view

One of the unsung benefits of Yoga may be conceiving a baby when stress is the root cause of infertility. One memorable example of this idea is my (Larry's) students Dave and Adrian Lopez. Immersed in busy, demanding careers, they gave up Yoga. When they later decided to start a family, they tried unsuccessfully for three years to conceive despite repeated attempts and the best medical methods available to them. Their physician finally suggested that perhaps their fertility problems were stress related and that they practice Yoga together — which they did. Sounds hard to believe, but after 30 days of practice, which included my weekly class and general conditioning DVD (flip to the appendix), Adrian became pregnant. She continued her Yoga practice until her eighth month and later gave birth to a big, beautiful baby boy.

We don't recommend starting any new fitness regime, Hatha Yoga included, in the middle of a pregnancy. Conscious yogic relaxation and meditation, on the other hand, are right at any stage of your pregnancy, and may be helpful tools for labor as well. Your body, mind, and baby will be grateful to you!

Enjoying Yoga support as you — and the baby — grow

Pregnancy entails major physiological and psychological changes. Apart from modifying your shape and weight, it also alters your body chemistry. Thus, you may experience a range of discomforts as well as the welcome feelings of anticipation, excitement, and joy.

Yoga can make a major difference in your pregnancy experience. The increased self-awareness that Yoga brings is very helpful during this special time when your body is continually undergoing change. Yogic practice provides the many benefits during that special time in your — and your baby's — life. Yoga

- ✔ Relaxes your whole body

- ✔ Helps with back problems

- ✔ Relieves nausea

- ✔ Reduces swelling and leg cramps

- ✔ Improves mood

- ✔ Provides focusing and breathing techniques for labor

- ✔ Provides a sense of community and social support through prenatal and postnatal Yoga classes

When seeking out prenatal Yoga classes, talk to the teacher beforehand. Ask about her training and experience and assure yourself that she's knowledgeable about modifications that would be safe and helpful during pregnancy.

Exercising caution during pregnancy

Because pregnancy is a time when your actions directly and immediately affect you and your developing baby, we recommend that you keep the following cautions in mind as you exercise:

- Always do a little less than you're used to doing, and never hold your breath.

- Stay away from extremes in all the postures, especially deep forward or back bends. Don't strain.

- Avoid lying on your stomach for any postures.

- Steer clear of sit-ups and postures that put pressure on the uterus.

- Skip the postures that solely focus on tightening the abs; rather, work on strengthening your core in the context of more gentle postures.

- When a posture calls for a twist, twist from the shoulders and not the belly to avoid compressing the internal organs.

- Avoid inverted postures other than putting your feet up on the wall or a chair.

- Pass up breathing exercises that are jarring, such as the shining skull *(kapala-bhati)* or breath of fire *(bhastrika).*

- Don't jump or move quickly in and out of postures.

✔ Be careful not to overstretch, which you can easily do in pregnancy because of increased hormone levels that cause your joints to become very limber.

 ACOG recommends that a pregnant woman avoid lying on her back during exercise — and that includes Yoga.

Perfect Pregnancy Postures

Practicing Yoga during pregnancy calls for the same consideration as putting together a yogic plan to manage back problems — no single posture or routine works the same way for everyone. Plus, what feels right during one trimester may not be appropriate during the next. In general, postures that allow you to gently increase flexibility in your hips should be useful as you prepare for giving birth, and a number of postures achieve that safely. We recommend you seek out a qualified Yoga teacher to guide you in either a prenatal Yoga class or one-on-one instruction.

In the following sections, we describe three of the most recommended and useful Yoga postures for you to use any time during pregnancy and postpartum. We also describe a safe 15-to-20 minute Yoga routine that helps relieve discomforts and prepare your body for childbirth.

Side-lying posture

Use the side-lying posture as an alternative to the corpse posture *(shavasana)* in your practice. You may also want to use the posture on its own to relieve feelings of general fatigue or nausea during pregnancy, labor, and the postpartum period, or as a good position for nursing. You need four or five blankets or three large pillows.

1. **Lie on your side on a comfortable surface.**

2. **Place one of the pillows or blankets under your head and the other just in front of you on the floor between the top of your thighs and the bottom of your chest.**

   Hang your top arm over the pillow in front of you.

3. **Bend your knees and place two blankets between your feet and your knees (see Figure 16-1).**

Figure 16-1:
Side-lying posture.

Stay and breathe naturally for as long as you feel comfortable. Repeat as often as you need to.

The cat and cow

This posture, a variation of the cat *(chakravakasana)*, extends the lower back and helps relieve symptoms of general back pain caused by pregnancy.

Don't exaggerate or force your lower back down in Step 4. Don't practice this pose if you experience any negative symptoms.

1. **Starting on your hands and knees, look straight ahead.**

2. **Place your knees at hip width and your hands below your shoulders.**

   Straighten your elbows, but don't lock them.

3. **As you exhale, arch your back like a cat.**

   Turn your head down and look at the floor (see Figure 16-2a).

4. **As you inhale, slowly look up toward the ceiling and drop your lower back, so that the shape of your back resembles that of a cow, as shown in Figure 16-2b.**

5. **Repeat Steps 3 and 4 six to eight times.**

Figure 16-2: *The cat and cow.*

The cobbler's posture: Badda konasana

The cobbler's posture helps you prepare for delivery by opening your groin and hips. It also improves alignment and provides a sitting posture for advanced breathing (remember — no holding your breath) and meditation techniques.

1. **Sit on the floor with your legs straight out in front of you.**

   Place your hands palms down at your sides with your fingers forward.

2. **Shake your legs out in front of you a few times.**

3. **Bend your knees outward and slide the soles of your feet towards each other until they touch.**

   Hold the sides of your feet and lift gently up from the chest (see Figure 16-3).

Figure 16-3:
The cobbler's posture.

Sit in the posture for 30 seconds to a minute; as you progress, you can gradually increase to 3 to 5 minutes.

If your knees aren't close to the floor you can sit on blankets or place the blankets under your knees.

A safe, quick prenatal routine

The short routine in this section includes postures that are safe throughout pregnancy and focuses on the areas of the body that you want to strengthen as you prepare your body for giving birth. Chapter 7 gives you more information on these postures.

Mountain posture: Tadasana

One of the benefits of the mountain posture during pregnancy is that it directs your attention to your posture during this period when your weight and balance have gradually but steadily changed.

After you find your center of balance, begin the process of making a mental shift (which we discuss in Chapter 14), using the breathing style of your choice from Chapter 5. Stay in mountain posture (as shown in Figure 16-4) for 6 to 8 breaths.

Figure 16-4:
Mountain
posture.

Warrior I: Vira bhadrasana I

As its name may suggest, warrior I strengthens the legs and improves stamina and balance. It's especially beneficial during pregnancy because it stretches your hips and helps with tension in your neck and swelling in your fingers.

Move in and out of the posture 3 to 4 times and then stay for 6 to 8 breaths on each side. Figure 16-5 illustrates.

Figure 16-5:
Warrior I.

Warrior II: Vira bhadrasana II

Another variation in the warrior family, this powerful posture opens your hips as it builds stamina and strengthens your arms. Move in and out of the posture 3 to 4 times and then stay for 6 to 8 breaths on each side. Check out Figure 16-6.

Figure 16-6:
Warrior II.

Standing spread-legged forward bend: Prasarita pada uttanasana

This modified forward bend improves circulation in the

head and lengthens the spine, hamstrings, and adductor muscles on the inside of the thighs. Just hang in this posture (shown in Figure 16-7) for 6 to 8 breaths.

You can also try this standing posture with your hips at a wall or door.

Figure 16-7:
Standing spread-legged forward bend.

Triangle posture: Utthita trikonasana

The triangle posture stretches the sides of the spine, the back of the legs, and the hips while it opens the chest. Move in and out of the posture 3 to 4 times and then stay for 6 to 8 breaths on each side. Figure 16-8 gives you a visual.

Figure 16-8:
Triangle posture.

Supported chair squatting posture: Modified ardha utkatasana

The supported chair builds overall stamina while it strengthens your back, legs, shoulders, and arms. Move in and out of the posture 3 to 4 times and then stay for 6 to 8 breaths.

Use an actual chair as illustrated in Figure 16-9 unless you feel comfortable without it. Use a wide stance to maintain your center of balance.

Figure 16-9:
Supported chair squatting posture.

Use your Yoga tools to ease your labor — and have a healthier child

In their pure and hybrid forms, all the various methods of childbirth preparation — Lamaze, The Bradley Method, Birthing from Within, Birthworks, and Hypnobirthing — draw upon techniques that are integral to Yoga. In its own way, each method teaches the laboring woman to focus on her breath, breathe into a focal point, and/or utilize relaxation and meditation techniques. Your Yoga practice can help you more effectively utilize whichever method of childbirth preparation you choose. Why is this connection important when the pain of childbirth can be controlled pharmacologically? Because babies born through nonmedicated births are better able to breastfeed, and breastfed babies are healthier, as are their mothers. You and your baby may continue to reap the benefits of your prenatal Yoga practice through your lifetimes.

Cobbler's posture

This posture (flip to "The cobbler's posture" and Figure 16-3 earlier in this chapter) is a wonderfully relaxing way to end this short routine. Use an advanced breathing technique from Chapter 5, such as alternate nostril breathing, that doesn't require breath retention, and/or a meditation technique from Chapter 21.

Continuing Yogic Exercise after Pregnancy (Postpartum)

Many traditional cultures honor a period of rest for the newly delivered mother to give her time to recover from childbirth and bond with her newborn. This break typically lasts about four to six weeks; in Spanish, it's known as *la cuarentena,* or "the 40-day quarantine." Not surprisingly, physicians generally recommend that new mothers wait about six weeks before resuming their usual exercise routines, and a couple of weeks longer if they had a Caesarean section.

When you return to your Yoga mat, avoid all inverted postures for at least six weeks postpartum because of uterine blood flow (called *lochia*). Also, be careful with sit-ups because the groin area is fragile from its recent stretch. A good way to get started is with short walks and the side-lying corpse posture (see "Side-lying posture" and Figure 16-1 earlier in the chapter). All women have postnatal bleeding for a few weeks after pregnancy. Watch your flow and slow down your Yoga practice a little if the bleeding becomes heavier or turns bright red. If in doubt, consult your physician.

If you can, seek out a postpartum class with other new mothers. A skilled and experienced Yoga teacher can focus on those areas of your body that are likely to need extra attention during this transitional period — neck, shoulders, and upper back from the stress of carrying your baby and leaning over to attend to him or her; gentle belly toners to help you regain your pre-pregnancy profile; and so on. And don't underestimate the value of connecting with other new mothers. Few new mothers are fully prepared for the feelings of isolation and lack of control over their daily lives that are so common in the early postpartum period, especially among women who are used to being in the world and getting things done. The company of other new mothers who are feeling similar things is often comforting and grounding.

Expect your life to change radically after the baby is born.

Your Yoga practice will seem like an oasis, even if your practice sessions are short, as you handle the joyful but exhausting responsibilities of caring for your new baby. Don't feel guilty about making and taking time for yourself. You need to recharge. Your hormone levels may make you feel emotional and a little unstable, and your Yoga practice can help you find balance. Final relaxation after your postures helps you feel more rested even though the enjoyment of a full night's sleep may be but a sweet and distant memory.

Your child took nine months to grow inside your body, so give yourself nine months to get back into shape. Set your clock to "mommy time" and enjoy the ride.

Chapter 17

Yoga for Kids and Teens

• •

In This Chapter

▶ Understanding how to make Yoga fun and safe for kids
▶ Trying some kid-friendly poses
▶ Easing the stress of adolescence with Yoga
▶ Checking out challenging Yoga routines perfect for teens and young adults

• •

Young people have a natural affinity for Yoga. You can introduce even the youngest children to Yoga through play. As the names of common Yoga postures reveal, the postures were inspired by animals — the cat, the cow, the dog, the bear, and so on. The focused coordination of movement and breath that makes these movements Yoga and not just physical exercise easily lends itself to child's play. When combined with play — for example, imitation of animals sounds, a magic box of plush animal toys, balls of various sizes — voilà! You have the beginnings of kid-friendly Yoga.

For the "young and restless," also known as teens, Yoga

offers tools to cultivate health in body, mind, and spirit. It provides a noncompetitive way for young people to develop strength and confidence, and manage stress — the plague of the times.

Classroom teachers are catching on to how Yoga can help their students gather up their boundless energy and focus on their academic tasks. Parents and Yoga teachers alike are finding that Yoga can also play a therapeutic role for children with challenges such as autism and ADHD.

In this chapter, we give pointers, sample postures, and kid-friendly ways for parents to introduce Yoga to their children. Teachers reading this book can find information here to whet their appetites for incorporating Yoga into their classrooms (resources are included in the appendix). Teens and adults with energy to spare also get a guide to a classical routine that challenges the body while focusing the mind.

Kid Stuff: Making Yoga Fun for Youngsters

The sense of calm, focus, and balance that draws adults to the practice of Yoga is also available to children, even those as young as three, as long as you introduce them to it in a playful, child-friendly fashion. When guided with a developmentally appropriate approach, preschoolers and the primary school set alike can reap Yoga's numerous benefits, such as improved concentration skills, an ability to calm and center themselves, and greater self-esteem and self-confidence. In many ways, young children are naturals for Yoga because they can participate without the physical and mental tightness that adults have acquired. Afi Kobari, creator of the *Yogamama* program in Los Angeles, describes a palpable energy and joy in her young students when she guides them through postures with a playful approach. The following sections give you some tips on engaging your child in Yoga, as well as several poses to try.

Engaging the imagination: Approaching poses in a child-friendly way

Child's play, when slowed down and joined with consciousness, can provide a platform for kid-friendly Yoga practice. Yoga postures (originally derived from and often named for animals) and concepts lend themselves to play in a variety of ways:

- Try having your child vocalize a posture's animal's call to draw attention to the breath.

- Let your child pick from selection of animal cards and then strike the pose of the chosen animal.

- Incorporate balance into any number of children's games that involve running and stopping at a specified moment by directing your child to be still and balance on one leg after stopping.

- Adding a children's Yoga book or idea with a story also helps to keep kids focused and share more philosophy with them in addition to asana.

- Add rolling a ball with one hand while the child's other hand is engaged in a seated posture to encourage right/left brain development.

Be flexible when introducing your child to Yoga. Keep the following pointers in mind:

- Short, happy practice sessions that your child wants to come back to are better than a longer session that loses her attention.

Bring balance to children with special needs

According to the Mayo Clinic, growing evidence suggests that Yoga may help alleviate symptoms of ADHD. On its physical level, Yoga encourages focus on breath before, during, and between postures, physical exertion through the *asanas,* and a focused winding down period afterwards, all of which can help calm your hyperactive tot. Yoga helps hyperactive children get in touch with their bodies in a relaxed and noncompetitive way, and its cumulative effects for your little yogi or yogini may result in improvements in their capacity for schoolwork and creative play. Seek out a Yoga teacher who can create a strong bond with your child to gain his trust and attention.

Yoga can also help children with autism gain new motor, communication, and social skills and thus enjoy an overall improvement in their quality of life. Structure and repetition are key for Yoga sessions for a child with autism. By gradually adding subtle modifications to the postures, one at a time, Yoga can help your child practice becoming comfortable with change. Over time, your little yogi or yogini develops a greater capacity to handle the stress that so often accompanies autism, along with greater body awareness and concentration.

The right Yoga teacher for your child with autism is someone who is respectful of her abilities as well as her challenges. This special teacher must be willing to meet your child where she is and gain her trust.

Be willing to adjust the Yoga session to your child's mood. A tired child may enjoy sitting poses. Cooling breathing exercises help a cranky child calm down. On a rainy day, active poses bring physical release of pent up energy.

Yoga postures kids will love

Children should skip the headstand and shoulder stand. Although their bodies are flexible, they lack the strength and stability to do those postures safely.

We designed the postures in the following sections to be kid-friendly and wrote the accompanying text to be parent-friendly as you guide your child. You can find more detail about each of the postures in other chapters throughout the book, as we note in each section; when done in sequence, this set of postures forms a well-balanced routine. In addition to providing you with instructions to give your child as he gets into the posture, the sections suggest sounds he can make while in the pose. The sounds serve a dual purpose: They inspire your child's imagination while he's holding the pose (keeping him engaged) and also guide him to breathe rather than hold his breath.

Note: In these sections, we sometimes refer to *yummy poses.* The term *yummy pose* is just a kid-friendly description of a resting pose, where you allow your body and mind to release. It was coined by Afi Kobari, a specialist in Yoga for children.

Children have short attention spans. You know your child best, so do only as many postures as he has attention for. In time, he'll be able to do more.

Find a special spot to practice Yoga with your child. Is there somewhere in your house or apartment where he gravitates to for play? That may be the perfect place to begin to share your love of Yoga.

The mountain posture

Figure 17-1 gives you and your child a visual of this kiddie posture; flip to Chapter 7 for more info on the adult version. Give your child the following instructions:

1. **Stand tall like a mountain.**

2. **Breathe through your nose and imagine you're in a very, very quiet place.**

Figure 17-1:
The mountain posture for kids.

Warrior I

See the preceding section for instructions to help get your child into mountain posture. Figure 17-2 and Chapter 7 give you more guidance on warrior I.

How long should your child hold a posture?

Younger children may only want to stay for a few seconds before they're ready to move. Older children can stay longer. Adults usually hold a position for six breaths after first having moved in and out of it a few times. Ask your child to hold the position only as long as you feel she will be comfortable. If she starts to get squirmy, have her come out of the position.

If your child's knee bends so much that you see it extending farther than the ankle, tell him to bend the knee a little bit less. The following instructions can lead your little yogi to warrior I success:

1. **Start in the mountain posture and take a big step forward with one leg.**

2. **Bend your front knee and raise your arms overhead by your ears.**

3. **Feel how powerful and strong you are in this posture; next time, as you bend your knee and raise your arms, say "Yes! I Can!"**

4. **Keeping your knee bent and your arms raised, stay in this position and really feel like a warrior.**

5. **Try the same movements on the other side.**

Figure 17-2:
Warrior I
for kids.

Bear posture

Check out Figure 17-3 and the following instructions to direct your child into bear posture.

1. **Start in the mountain posture and then bend forward and hang down.**

2. **Staying bent, walk around, dragging your arms and hands as you growl, and imagine you're a bear.**

Figure 17-3:
Bear posture for kids.

Cat and cow

The following directions help you walk your child through cat and cow; kids usually have a lot fun with this sequence, especially when you do it with them.

1. **Get down on your hands and knees as if you're going to crawl, but stay in one place.**

2. **Make your back round so you can look down and back at your legs.**

    Figure 17-4a illustrates this step.

3. **Imagine you're a cat and make the sound of a cat: meow.**

4. **Move your back so that your belly goes down towards the floor, your chest goes up, and you**

look ahead.

Show your child Figure 17-4b if he has trouble visualizing this step.

5. **Imagine you're a cow and make the sound of a cow: mooo, mooo.**

Figure 17-4:
Cat and cow posture for kids.

Jumping frog

Use these instructions to lead your tot through jumping frog:

1. **Stand with your feet wide apart and squat down low.**

   See Figure 17-5.

2. **Place your hands on the ground and then jump up and raise your arms.**

3. **Imagine you're a frog and make the sound of a frog: ribbit, ribbit.**

Figure 17-5:
Jumping frog for kids.

Tree posture

Work your child through tree posture by using the following instructions, and check out Figure 17-6 for an illustration. Flip to Chapter 7 for more information on the adult version.

1. **Start in the mountain posture, standing tall and still.**

2. **Bend one of your legs and place the bottom of that foot up high on the inside of the other thigh.**

3. **Bring your hands together up high above your head and imagine you're a tree, making the sound of the wind blowing through your leaves: shhhhhhh.**

4. **Now try the same movements on the other side.**

Figure 17-6:
Tree
posture for
kids.

Cobra II

Chapter 11 gives you more information on the adult version of cobra II; the following instructions and Figure 17-7 can help you lead your child through this version.

1. **Lie flat on your belly and place your hands on the floor near your armpits with your fingers going forward.**

2. **Raise your head, shoulders, and back as you press down on your hands, keeping your hips on the ground.**

3. **Imagine you're a cobra and make the cobra's sound: sssssss.**

Figure 17-7:
Cobra II for
kids.

Lion posture

With the help of these instructions and Figure 17-8, your youngster can take pride in her lion posture. (Chapter 6 provides additional information on the adult version.)

1. **Sit on your heels and place your hands on your knees.**

2. **Open your mouth wide, stick your tongue way out, and roll your eyes upward as though you're trying to see something high above you.**

3. **Imagine you're a mighty lion and roar: ahhaahh!**

Figure 17-8:
Lion posture
for kids.

Downward-facing dog

We discuss the adult version of this posture in Chapter 7, but the following steps and Figure 17-9 lay out a child-friendly variety.

1. **Start on your hands and knees.**

2. **Press through your arms, pushing down on your hands; straighten your legs and look down.**

3. **Imagine you're a dog and bark: woof, woof.**

Figure 17-9:
Downward-
facing dog
for kids.

Child's posture

This pose (one of the yummy poses) even has *child* in the name! Use the following instructions and Figure 17-10 to guide your tyke through child's posture.

1. **Kneel on the ground and fold up like a ball.**

2. **Place your hands at your sides with your palms up.**

3. **Relax and think good thoughts.**

The bridge

Figure 17-11 illustrates this easy posture; give your child the following instructions to help her through the pose, and check out Chapter 14 for the adult bridge.

1. **Lie on your back, bending your knees and letting your feet be firm on the ground.**

2. **Place your arms at your sides with your palms down.**

3. **Raise your hips up and become a bridge.**

4. **Imagine you're a bridge and make the sound of the cars traveling over you: chuga chuga chuga.**

Figure 17-10:
Child's posture for kids.

Figure 17-11:
Bridge for kids.

The wheel

The following directions and Figure 17-12 help your child get rolling with the wheel posture.

This advanced posture requires a fair amount of strength and flexibility. If your child isn't ready for it, wait until she becomes stronger and more flexible and come back to it.

1. **Lie on your back with your knees bent and your feet on the ground.**

2. **Place your arms over your head and turn your hands so that they're flat and your fingers are facing back towards your head.**

3. **Press up into the wheel.**

4. **Smile from the inside out.**

Figure 17-12:
Wheel for kids.

Knee-hugger

Knee-hugger is another of the yummy poses. These steps and Figure 17-13 show you how to help your child do it. You can find the adult version in Chapter 14 (though there it's called "knees-to-chest").

 For an added benefit have your child rock his knees from side to side while he's hugging them — it gently massages the back.

1. **Lie on your back and then bend and hug in your knees.**

2. **Just relax and think good thoughts.**

Figure 17-13:
Knee hugger for kids.

372

Easy posture

These instructions help you walk (sit?) your young yogini through easy posture; check out Figure 17-14 for the proper sitting posture. (We cover the adult version in Chapter 6.)

Your child may be more comfortable with a blanket under her hips.

1. **Sit on the floor and cross your legs comfortably.**

2. **Keep your back and head tall without straining.**

3. **Imagine a big balloon in your belly: When you breathe in, fill the balloon, and when you breathe out, let the air out of the balloon.**

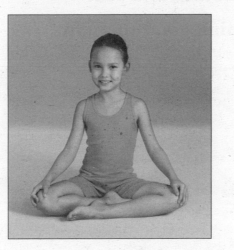

Figure 17-14:
Easy posture for kids.

The big yummy posture: Shavasana

Use the following instructions to help your child relax at the end of the session. Figure 17-15 illustrates the pose, and you can read more about the adult version in Chapter 4.

1. **Lie flat on your back, turning your palms up**

and letting your feet flop out.

2. **Close your eyes gently or keep them open and soft — whichever feels best.**

3. **Relax and think good thoughts.**

Figure 17-15: Shavasana for kids.

Easing the Transition into Adulthood: Yoga for Teens

Yoga practice in the teenage years is so much more than an exercise program. Yes, it provides an energy outlet and a way to build muscle and flexibility — both important in their own right. But Yoga practice also provides you with an entry point for a healthful and balanced perspective on life and themselves that can serve for a lifetime. The follow-

Integrating Yoga into the classroom

The lessons of Yoga aren't confined to the Yoga mat or the body. The skills and understanding acquired through Yoga practice help children of all ages, including teens, approach life in a more grounded, centered, and emotionally intelligent way. When presented as an exploration, traditional Yoga themes such as the practice of *ahimsa,* or non-harming (see Chapter 20), can be translated into simple, practical distinctions, such as the difference between force and finesse. Take the simple exercise of untying a knot: By using finesse rather than force, a child learns through his own experience which is the better way. This awareness applied to Yoga poses and balance allows a child to recognize which feels best in his own body; applied to personal relationships, it illustrates the better way to get along with the people in his life.

You don't need to be a Yoga teacher to bring this often-neglected aspect of learning into the classroom. Classroom teachers can learn to lead children through basic poses and routines to enhance their ability to learn throughout the day — for instance, morning sun salutations (see Chapter 14) to energize and focus their energy; balancing poses (see Chapter 9) after recess to regroup for academics; alternate nostril breathing (see Chapter 5) in a comfortable seated pose (see Chapter 7) or a simple forward bend (see Chapter 12) to help calm the mind as a prelude to creative writing. The list goes on. To date, over 1,000 schools have integrated Yoga techniques into their curricula through the training and materials available through Yoga Playgrounds and Yoga Ed, both developed by Leah Kalish.

ing sections describe some benefits Yoga can offer teens.

The antidote to stress in your overscheduled life

Maybe you're vying for a place on the team or a high class ranking, juggling a part-time job, or caring for younger siblings while being a full-time student. More likely than not, your time and energy are stretched to the max.

And your shifting hormonal levels may leave you feeling like a different person from day to day, hour to hour, and even minute to minute.

Yoga can be an oasis in a vast desert of stress. Yoga, a union of mind and body, can make weathering the demands of daily life easier. With regular practice, you may find that you have a greater ability to think for yourself and trust yourself — important at a time of life when peer pressure can feel overwhelming and poor judgment and bad decisions can impact your health, well-being, and your future.

Headstands, shoulder stands, and the lotus position may look like the popular idea of Yoga, but in fact they can be dangerous. Young people who are still growing don't yet have the necessary musculature and stability to tackle these postures safely, so stay away from them for the time being.

Fit for life, and so much more

Perhaps the most important benefit Yoga can offer you as a teen is the opportunity to develop a lifelong friendship with your body. When you develop a Yoga practice, first under the guidance of a skilled and nurturing teacher and then later on your own, you tune in to your body, pay attention to what's happening, and respond appropriately — not unlike the good energy you put into your friendships with your best buddies. A regular Yoga practice can help you develop the focus, concentration, and discipline you need to study well and pursue your dreams. And when you're barefooted on your mat in the practice studio, you're free from the pecking order of your school campus. Yoga helps you become self confident and courageous, without competing. How good is that?

Of course, Yoga is also a great way to become and stay fit. Both the USDA and Health Canada rank having an adequate level of physical activity as a high health priority. The revised USDA Food Pyramid (www.mypyramid.gov) actually includes it as part of a balanced diet.

As a form of physical fitness, Yoga is an attractive package:

- It's economical. You already have this book, so you can begin practicing right away without anything else.

- You don't need a gym or a playing field. You just need enough floor space to practice safely. If you practice at home, try to find a private space. If your space is at a premium, consider following the lead of a highly-respected Yoga teacher who's been known to practice "bathroom Yoga" when no other private space was available. Building codes require even the smallest bathrooms to have a certain amount of floor space. Check it out. Yours may just be long enough for a mat.

Can Yoga help you maintain a healthy weight?

According to Robert M. Sapolsky's *Why Zebras Don't Get Ulcers* (Henry Holt and Company), modern garden variety stressors can lead to overeating, and in particular, choosing the wrong kinds of food to overeat. Stress floods your body with hormones that affect your appetite. If the stress is intense but short-lived, most people usually experience a loss of appetite — the way you feel when you're too nervous to eat. But when you experience frequent on-and-off stress throughout the course of the day, day in and day out, the hormonal levels in the body increase appetite — and not for the healthy stuff. What helps? Regular exercise that you look forward to doing, meditation, and cultivating a self-accepting, non-perfectionist approach to life are a few things that have been shown to help. How handy to be able to find all of that in Yoga.

Yoga Routines for the Young and Restless

The routines in this section have been specifically designed for teens. When done carefully, they also work for men and women well into their 30s, but we don't recommend them for the typical middle-aged person over 40. A lot of what group Yoga classes across America (especially in health clubs) offer today was originally designed for lightweight teenage boys in India whose lifestyles involved a lot of squatting. Middle-aged beginners often jump into that kind of Yoga in a competitive way and end up with injuries to show for it because it's just not built for them (or they for it).

Most professional athletes are usually at their highest physical prowess from their teens to early 30s. Then the body starts to change, and so should the training program to prevent injuries. I (Larry) call the first stage "Yoga for the Young and Restless." Many of the popular styles of Yoga, such as Ashtanga Yoga, some components of Iyengar Yoga, and modern flow Yoga, were inspired by the teachings of the late Sri T. Krishnamacharya of Southern India earlier in his life, and were originally intended for younger practitioners. The unpublished routines in this section were passed down to me (Larry) by Sri T. Krishnamacharya's son (and my teacher) T.K.V. Desikachar.

These routines are meant to be challenging. However, always keep in mind Yoga's fundamental principle: "Do no harm." Trust your inner teacher. If your body says it's time to rest, rest (even if others are still in their poses). Trusting yourself in this way is an important step towards becoming a balanced adult.

Standing routine

As you get ready to begin your routine, remember that Yoga is a body, breath, and mind discipline. With the exception of the jumps, move slowly and stay in the moment.

Before you begin, here are some general tips and instructions to keep in mind:

- ✔ Choose either focus or chest-to-belly breathing from Chapter 5.

- ✔ Stay and breathe in each posture for 8 to 10 breaths.

- ✔ Do the whole routine twice on both sides.

- ✔ Refer to Chapter 7 for detailed instruction on all the postures in this routine (though note that some postures here are variations on Chapter 7's postures).

✔ This routine should take about 15 to 20 minutes.

When you're ready, follow these steps to complete the standing routine:

1. **Start in the mountain posture (see Figure 17-16a).**

   Initiate the Yoga breathing style of your choice from the list earlier in this section.

2. **As you exhale, jump or step out into a wide stance with your arms in a *T* parallel to the floor as shown in Figure 17-16b.**

3. **As you inhale, raise your arms from the sides up and overhead as you rotate your feet and torso to the right as Figure 17-16c illustrates.**

4. **As you exhale, sink into warrior I position with your right knee bent in a 90-degree angle (like in Figure 17-16d).**

5. **As you inhale, rotate your shoulders to the left and drop your arms into a *T* with your palms down for the warrior II position.**

   Open your back (left) hip to the left as far as it can go and tuck your tail under comfortably. Figure 17-16e gives you a visual.

6. **As you exhale, rotate your shoulders to the right and reach forward with your left arm and back with your right arm so that they're parallel to the floor (as in Figure 17-16f) for the reverse triangle variation I.**

7. **Inhale and then, as you exhale, drop your left hand down to the floor and bring your right arm straight up for the reverse triangle**

variation II, keeping your right leg bent and rotating your head up to the right as shown in Figure 17-16g.

If your neck gets tired, turn your head down.

8. As you exhale, roll down with your arms, trunk, and head; turn your feet forward and parallel and then hang down the middle, holding your elbows for the standing spread-legged forward bend shown in Figure 17-16h.

9. Roll your body up and then jump or step back into the mountain posture in Step 1.

10. Repeat Steps 1 through 9 on the left side.

Figure 17-16:
Sequence of poses for the standing routine for teens.

Floor routine

Some people call this routine the Lifetime Sequence because getting into wide-legged seated forward bend postures takes a lifetime if you aren't naturally flexible in the hips. The beauty of Yoga is that if you don't achieve your goal in this lifetime, you can get there in the next.

Before you begin, here are some tips to keep in mind:

- ✔ Choose focus or chest-to-belly breathing from Chapter 5.

- ✔ Stay in each posture (including each time you raise your arms) for 6 to 8 breaths.

- ✔ Do the whole sequence twice.

- ✔ This routine should take 20 to 25 minutes.

- ✔ Feel free to soften your knees in all of the forward bends.

- ✔ Challenge yourself, but don't strain yourself.

 This routine isn't recommended for people with lower back problems aggravated by rounding.

When you're ready, follow these steps to complete the floor routine:

1. **Start with your arms in the air and a straight back as in Figure 17-17a.**

2. **As you exhale, bend forward and down to the seated forward bend pose shown in Figure 17-17b.**

3. **As you inhale, raise your trunk and arms up to a straight back and separate your legs wide like in Figure 17-17c.**

4. **As you exhale, bend forward and down to a spread-legged forward bend as Figure 17-17d illustrates.**

5. **As you inhale, raise your trunk and arms up to a straight back position as you did in Step 3**

383

(see Figure 17-17c).

6. As you exhale, rotate to the right as in Figure 17-17e and bend forward and down as shown in Figure 17-17f.

7. As you inhale, raise your trunk and arms up to a straight back position like you did in Step 5 (see Figure 17-17c).

8. As you exhale, rotate to the left like in Figure 17-17g and bend forward and down (see Figure 17-17h).

9. As you inhale, raise your trunk and arms up to a straight back position and bend your legs half way with your toes up as depicted in Figure 17-17i.

10. As you exhale, bend forward and down and try to move your toes down like in Figure 17-17j.

11. As you inhale, raise your trunk and arms up to a straight back position, drop your knees down to the sides and join the soles of your feet together as Figure 17-17k illustrates.

12. As you exhale, bend forward and down and hold your feet (see Figure 17-17l).

Figure 17-17:
Sequence of poses for the floor routine for teens.

 If you have back problems lifting up from the forward bends in this routine, try the "Roll Up": Keep your chin down on your chest and roll up, stacking the vertebrae one at a time, with your arms hanging at your sides. When you're fully upright, bring the arms up and overhead from the front and look forward.

Chapter 18

It's Never Too Late: Yoga for Midlifers and Older Adults

If you're on the senior side of the life curve and considering taking up Yoga, you're not alone. A 2008 *Yoga Journal* study reported that of the almost 16 million Americans who practice Yoga, almost 3 million are 55 or older.

Yoga can help practitioners of every age improve their health and well-being. The Yoga toolbox includes innumerable postures that, depending on how you modify them, can offer the appropriate level of challenge to each and every yogi and yogini regardless of age or ability. Remember, the process and the practice are what are important, not the final form of the postures. One advantage that more mature practitioners of Yoga have over its more youthful adherents is greater patience to be still for breathing exercises and meditation, both of which become more important relative to the postures as you age.

This chapter discusses and presents safe Yoga routines for people in their middle-aged and senior years. The Prime of Life Yoga discussion addresses folks who fall within the vast expanse of the middle years — generally between 40-something and 70-something.

The "Cherish the Chair" section addresses the needs of folks who are generally older than 70; however, these routines may be used and enjoyed by people of any age. Yoga is a union of body, breath, and mind, and that the best variations of Yoga postures for any individual are those that meet his or her own physical, emotional, and lifestyle needs regardless of age.

Reaping the Benefits of Yoga Through Midlife and Beyond

Midlife, as the word suggests, refers to the middle of life. It's not, as some people think, The End but rather a new beginning. The following sections show you how Yoga helps you navigate the physical and emotional changes associated with midlife and allows you to age gracefully, healthfully, and actively.

Working through menopause

Menopause signals a major biochemical change in a woman, marked most obviously by the disappearance of her monthly flow. Her body's sexual glands go into relative retirement, and she can no longer bear children. The hormonal shifts that lead up to the actual menopause may take up to a decade. *Perimenopause,* the term given to the longer process, can bring with it a host of undesirable side effects: hot flashes, palpitations, dizzy spells, insomnia, vaginal dryness, urinary problems, and irritability. This time of life can make women prone to depression, but with an attitude of acceptance for the change and the possibilities yet to come, it can actually be a very satisfying time of life. That's where Yoga comes in.

Regular Yoga practice can help alleviate the physiological side effects of menopause, especially if you start a few years before its onset, and help you cultivate a forgiving, accepting, and positive attitude important for your emotional well-being. Inversions (see Chapter 10), which have a profound effect on the glands and inner organs and literally and figuratively allow you to view things from a new perspective, are especially helpful. For soothing rest and whole-person recovery, we particularly recommend that you cultivate the corpse posture we describe in Chapter 15. Just give your body a chance to rebalance its chemistry.

Not just a "woman thing": Andropause

Men experience something similar to menopause called *andropause.* Although changes in their sexual glands may lessen their sex drives, men can continue to sire children into old age. But when they see their vitality and hairline recede a little, men are often thrown into an existential crisis.

Midlife offers a great opportunity to discover life's possibilities beyond sexual reproduction and raising children. Regular Yoga practice can buffer the unpleasant physiological side effects of andropause and stabilize the emotions that are triggered when you realize you're no longer quite so dashing — unless, of course, you have practiced Yoga all along.

Bones of steel

 With regular exercise, you can prevent the bone loss *(osteoporosis)* associated with midlife and old age. Regular weight-bearing exercises strengthen your bones, but stress causes acidity, which leaches the calcium from your bones. Many people don't realize that osteoporosis actually starts in your mid to late 20s. Therefore, you can't begin Yoga too early — and it's never too late to take it up! Buns of steel ain't bad, but bones of steel are the better deal.

Approaching Prime of Life Yoga with the Right Mindset

As you age, mobility is the new flexibility. So although you may have been able to do the most acrobatic postures in your youth, the important goal now is to maintain the mobility to remain fit and active. In the Prime of Life approach to Yoga postures, spinal freedom and movement take precedence over form. Adjustments to the posture, such as bending the knees a *lot* if necessary, encourage movement of the spine.

The attitude you bring to your practice is critical. The right attitude on the mat allows you to practice postures safely and spills over to your life off the mat. Here are a few Yoga principles for a safe and fulfilling practice.

- ✔ Challenge yourself but don't strain yourself.

- ✔ Yoga is a dialogue, not a monologue; keep body, breath, and mind linked.

- ✔ Think of your Yoga practice as a meditation in motion.

- ✔ You get no gain with *negative pain* (pain that does harm).

- ✔ You're the chairman of the board; you decide when to come out of the posture.

- ✔ Let the posture fit you instead of trying to fit yourself into the posture.

User-Friendly Routines for Midlifers

In this section, we present routines for two different skill levels, both of which are equally ideal for men and women. (For true beginners with a few aches or pains, we recommend starting with the lower back routine in Chapter 22.)

 You can find recommendations for DVDs on Yoga for this age group in the appendix.

Prime of Life Yoga routine: Level I

The routine described and illustrated in this section is a nice general-conditioning routine for midlifers and even younger folks who want to ease back into physical activity. This user-friendly sequence strings together a series of safe postures that work each side of the body separately, helping to achieve greater balance.

You can find detailed instructions for each of these various poses or their variations in Chapters 4, 7, 8, and 15. Choose a breathing technique from Chapter 5. Hold each posture and its variation for six to eight breaths, with the exception of warrior I (described in Steps 2 and 3) and revolved triangle variation (Steps 9 and 10). For each of these, move into and out of the postures three times and then hold for six to eight breaths. This routine should take about 30 to 35 minutes.

1. **Start in the mountain posture shown in Figure 18-1a.**

   Initiate the Yoga breathing style of your choice for six to eight breaths (see Chapter 5).

2. **As you exhale, step forward with the right foot about 3 to 3 1/2 feet (or the length of one leg).**

   Your left foot will turn out naturally. (Turn it out more to increase stability.) Place your hands on the tops of your hips and square the front of your pelvis; release your hands and hang your arms (see Figure 18-1b).

3. **As you inhale, raise your arms from the front up and overhead and bend your right leg into a right angle for warrior I as Figure 18-1c illustrates.**

4. **Repeat Steps 2 and 3 three times and then stay in warrior I for six to eight breaths.**

5. **As you exhale, bend both arms downward and draw your elbows back as you turn your palms up and lift your chest as shown in Figure 18-1d; hold this proud warrior posture for six to eight breaths.**

6. **As you inhale, keep your right leg bent; join your palms together in front of you and bring them up and overhead as you look up and back as in Figure 18-1e.**

Stay in the exalted warrior posture for six to eight breaths.

7. **As you exhale, come down over your bent right leg and place your hands on the floor for the standing asymmetrical forward bend as Figure 18-1f indicates; stay in the posture for six to eight breaths.**

   Work on straightening your right leg based on your flexibility in the moment. A soft or bent leg is okay.

   TIP If you want to feel the stretch more, square your hips by pulling the right hip back and the left hip forward. A more challenging option is to rotate the back foot inward, called *paralleling the feet.*

8. **As you inhale roll your body up vertebra by vertebra and then step your feet together back into the mountain posture from Step 1.**

9. **Repeat Steps 1 through 8 on the left side.**

10. **From the mountain posture, step out with your right foot about 3 to 3 1/2 feet (or the length of one leg); as you exhale, bend forward from the hips, hang down, and place the palms of both hands on the floor directly below your shoulders as shown in Figure 18-1g.**

11. **As you inhale, raise your right arm up towards the ceiling and look up at your right hand for the reverse triangle posture as Figure 18-1h illustrates.**

12. **Repeat Steps 10 and 11 three times and then remain with your right arm up for six to eight breaths.**

Soften your knees and arms. Turn your head down if your neck gets sore. Repeat on your left side.

13. **As you exhale, hang your torso, head, and arms down, holding your bent elbows with opposite-side hands for the standing spread-legged forward bend (see Figure 18-1i); stay for six to eight breaths.**

14. **Transition to your hands and knees and slide your right hand forward and your left leg back as you exhale, keeping your hand and your toes on the floor; as you inhale, raise your right arm and left leg to a comfortable height for the balancing cat posture as shown in Figure 18-1j.**

    Stay up for four to eight breaths and then repeat with opposite pairs, lifting your left hand and your right leg.

    If you want a bigger challenge in this posture, raise your bottom foot just off the floor.

15. **As you exhale, come back to all fours and fold down into the child's posture variation (with your arms in front of you) in Figure 18-1k; hold for six to eight breaths.**

16. **Lie flat on your back with your arms along the sides of your torso, your palms up, and your eyes closed for the corpse posture as in Figure 18-1l.**

17. **To finish, use belly breathing from Chapter 5 or a relaxation technique from Chapter 4 for three to five minutes.**

Figure 18-1:
Prime of Life Yoga routine: Level I.

Prime of Life Yoga routine: Level II

After you master the level I sequence described in the preceding section, enjoy the challenge of this section's level II sequence. It's a little longer and more physically demanding, and like the other routine, brings balance by working each side of the body separately.

Plan to spend approximately 45 minutes to complete this sequence, which is broken into two parts: standing postures and postures on the floor.

For detailed information on the various postures in this section or their variations, head to Chapters 4, 7, 8, 11, 12, and 15. Select a breathing technique from Chapter 5. Hold each posture and variation for six to eight breaths, with the exception of the warrior II posture (Steps 3 and 4), and the seated forward bend posture (Steps 12 and 13), both of which you move into and out of three times before holding for six to eight breaths.

1. **Start in the mountain posture illustrated in Figure 18-2a.**

   Initiate the Yoga breathing style of your choice from Chapter 5 for six to eight breaths.

2. **As you exhale, step out to your right with your right foot about 3 to 3 1/2 feet (or the length of one leg); turn your right foot out 90 degrees and your left foot inward 45 degrees.**

3. **As you inhale, raise your arms out to your sides in a *T* parallel to the line of your shoulders and the floor for the warrior II ready posture as Figure 18-2b indicates.**

4. **As you exhale, bend your right knee to a right angle with the floor and turn your head to the right as shown in Figure 18-2c; repeat Steps 3 and 4 three times and then remain in the warrior II posture for six to eight breaths.**

5. **As you inhale, raise your right arm and turn your right palm up; as you exhale, reach back**

with your left hand (palm down) and hold the outside of your left leg, looking up at your right hand for the reverse warrior posture (see Figure 18-2d), and stay for six to eight breaths.

6. As you inhale, move back briefly to the warrior II position and then bend your right arm, lay your right forearm across the top of your right thigh, and extend your left arm over your head in alignment with your left ear as illustrated in Figure 18-2e; stay in this extended right angle posture for six to eight breaths.

7. Repeat Steps 1 through 6 on the left side.

8. From your wide stance, roll your body up, turn both feet forward (to the right), and hang your arms at your sides; as you exhale, bend forward from the hips and hang your torso, head, and arms down, holding your bent elbows with opposite-side hands in the standing spread-legged forward bend as Figure 18-2f demonstrates for six to eight breaths.

9. Return to mountain posture (refer to Figure 18-2a).

10. As you inhale, raise your arms from the front up and overhead; as you exhale, bend forward from the hips, raise your left leg back and up until your arms, torso, and left leg are all parallel to the floor and you're balancing on your right leg in the warrior III posture. See Figure 18-2g for six to eight breaths.

11. Repeat Steps 9 and 10, balancing on the other side with your left leg.

Figure 18-2:
*Prime of Life
Yoga routine:
Level II, part 1.*

12. **Lie on your back with your knees bent and feet flat on the floor at hip width and place your hands at your sides palms down; as you inhale, raise your hips up and your arms overhead to touch the floor behind you in the bridge variation with arm raise posture as shown in Figure 18-3a for six to eight breaths.**

13. **Lie on your abdomen with your left arm forward (palm down) and your right arm back at your right side (palm up) and then bend your right knee and hold your right foot with your right hand, lifting your chest, left arm, and right foot to a comfortable level as you inhale into the half bow posture (see Figure 18-3b); stay up for six to eight breaths and then repeat with opposite pairs, holding your left**

foot with your left hand and extending your right arm forward.

14. **Move to your hands and knees with both at hip width; as you exhale, sit back on your heels and fold your head and hips down into a comfortable position for the child's posture variation as Figure 18-3c illustrates — stay folded for six to eight breaths.**

15. **Transition to a seated position with your legs stretched out in front of you and bring your back up nice and tall, moving your arms forward and up alongside your ears as you inhale, as demonstrated in Figure 18-3d.**

16. **As you exhale, bend forward from your hips, bringing your hands, chest, and head toward the floor as shown in Figure 18-3e; repeat Steps 15 and 16 three times and then stay down and folded for six to eight breaths.**

Soften your legs and arms as needed.

Take extra caution or avoid seated straight-legged forward bends if you have back problems that are exacerbated by rounding the back.

17. **Lie flat on your back with your legs stretched out and your arms extended out into a *T* with your palms up, and as you exhale, bring your right leg up and across your torso to the opposite side, slide your left arm overhead, and turn your head to the right until you are in the Swiss army knife as in Figure 18-3f; stay in the posture for six to eight breaths and then repeat with opposite pairs.**

Soften your limbs as needed.

Figure 18-3:
Prime of Life Yoga routine: Level II, part 2.

18. **Stay on your back and hug both your knees to your chest with your hands as you exhale for the knees-to-chest posture (see Figure 18-3g); hold for six to eight breaths.**

Hold on under your thighs if you have knee problems. As an alternative, rock gently from side to side.

19. **Lie flat on your back in the corpse posture (refer to Figure 18-2h) with your arms along the sides of your torso, your palms up, and your eyes closed to finish, use belly breathing from Chapter 5 or a relaxation technique from Chapter 4 for three to five minutes.**

Yoga for Older Adults

According to the National Institute on Aging (www.nia.nih. gov), "'Too old' and 'too frail' are not, in and of themselves, reasons to prohibit physical activity. In fact, there aren't very many health reasons to keep older adults from becoming more active." Rather, many chronic conditions are actually a result of *not* exercising. As a form of exercise, Yoga has many benefits that are specific to seniors. Improved balance and flexibility reduce the risk for (and fear of) injury and increase mobility. Yoga also improves circulation and your ability to sleep, and adding even light weights to the postures increases bone density and lowers the risk of fracture. Plus, group practice promotes social interaction and sense of connectedness.

Seniors interested in Yoga should first check with their physicians. After you get the green light, seek out a class that focuses on your age group both for the social benefits and to be guided by a teacher who is knowledgeable about adapting postures to your needs and abilities. Head to Chapter 2 for more on picking a teacher and a class. Be sure to mention any physical conditions or concerns (such as high blood pressure, hip replacement, osteoporosis, and so on) and verify whether your prospective teacher can modify the routines to ensure your safety. In a group setting, a skilled teacher offers a range of options so that each student can practice at a level appropriate for his or her abilities and limitations.

Cherish the Chair: Safe Routines for Older Adults

You don't have to practice Yoga on the floor. If getting down to the floor or getting up and down is difficult, chair

How old is too old for Yoga?

Shelly Kinney, a Las Vegas-based Yoga therapist, recounts her experience with Ms. L, a 96-year-old student who was glued to her walker. After several months of Yoga practice, Ms. L was able to enter and leave the class without it. How did this happen? She executed warrior and side angle postures from a chair, adding light weights over time, and worked with balance postures with a ballet bar on one side, a chair at the other, and Shelley there for support. Slowly but surely, Ms. L built up strength, flexibility, and confidence. She's proof that you're never too old to take up Yoga and enjoy its benefits.

Yoga offers spinal freedom while allowing you to remain in your comfort zone. You can improve your flexibility, mobility, and balance even while seated, and the following routines show you how.

You're in charge of whether or not you do a particular posture. If it doesn't feel right for you, don't do it. The National Institute on Aging provides a wealth of information to help guide you on what may be safe for you and what you should avoid. We also list books addressing the needs of older practitioners in the appendix, and your Yoga teacher may suggest other books or articles as well. Educate yourself, and enjoy the benefits of breath and movement.

Cherish the chair routine: Level I

The postures in this seated Yoga routine give you the same main benefits of a regular Yoga class, including stress reduction, improved circulation, better concentration and an overall sense of well-being. This routine should take about 15 to 20 minutes. Choose one of the Yoga breathing techniques in Chapter 5 and use it for this entire routine. Follow the instructions for breath and movement and have fun!

Place blankets or a block under your feet if they don't sit flat on the floor in any of the chair postures.

Seated mountain posture

Check out Figure 18-4 and the following steps for a visual of this posture.

1. **Sit comfortably in a chair with your back extended and your eyes either open or closed.**

2. **Hang your arms at your sides and visualize a vertical line down the middle of your ears, shoulders, hips, and the backs of your hands; stay for eight to ten breaths.**

Figure 18-4:
Seated mountain posture.

Seated mountain arm variation

You can see how it's done in Figure 18-5. Just follow these steps:

402

1. **Start in the seated mountain posture from the preceding section and raise your right arm and turn your head to the left as you inhale.**

2. **As you exhale, return to the seated mountain posture.**

3. **Repeat Steps 1 and 2 with your left arm and a right head turn, alternating right and left sides slowly for a total of 4 to 6 repetitions on each side.**

Figure 18-5:
Seated mountain posture variation.

Seated karate kid variation

Figure 18-6 illustrates this posture. Executing it is easy:

1. **Start in the seated mountain posture and raise your arms forward and up alongside of your ears as you inhale.**

2. **As you exhale, bend your right knee and raise it upward toward your chest to a comfortable level.**

3. **Take another breath and then, as you exhale,**

lower your right knee and your arms back to the seated mountain posture.

4. **Repeat Steps 1 through 3 with both arms and your left knee, alternating both of your knees slowly as you raise your arms for a total of 4 to 6 repetitions on each side.**

Be careful with this posture if you have a hip replacement. If you aren't sure whether your hips can handle it, check with your doctor first.

Figure 18-6:
Seated karate kid variation.

Seated wing-and-prayer

Figure 18-7 shows you this posture. Here's how you do it:

1. **Start in the seated mountain posture with your hands together in prayer position with your thumbs at your breastbone.**

2. **As you inhale, open your hands outward and lift your chest like wings.**

3. **As you exhale, bring your hands and arms back together into the prayer position.**

4. **Repeat Steps 1 through 3 slowly for 4 to 6 repetitions.**

Figure 18-7:
Seated wing-and-prayer.

Seated butterfly posture

Check out the seated butterfly in Figure 18-8 and then follow these steps to try it on your own.

1. **Start in the seated mountain posture with your arms extended out fully to the sides and parallel to the floor and your palms facing forward.**

2. **Inhale, and then as you exhale, bring your right hand towards the inside of your left arm in a twisting motion.**

3. **Repeat Steps 1 and 2 slowly for 4 to 6 repetitions and then do the same with your left hand and right arm.**

Figure 18-8:
*Seated
butterfly
posture.*

Standing warrior I chair variation

Use Figure 18-9 and the following steps to guide you through this posture.

1. **Stand in the mountain posture (see Figure 18-2a earlier in the chapter), facing the back of your chair from about 3 to 3 1/2 feet away.**

2. **As you exhale, step forward with your right leg, place your hands on the back of the chair, and bend your forward leg into approximately a right angle.**

   You can keep the back foot flat or pivot on the ball of the back foot. Don't be tempted to force the angle.

3. **Stay in Step 2 for 4 to 6 breaths and then repeat with your left leg forward for 4 to 6 breaths.**

Figure 18-9:
Standing warrior I chair variation.

Seated sage twist

Check out Figure 18-10 and the following steps for the seated sage twist.

1. **Sit in your chair sideways with the back of the chair to your right and your feet flat on the floor.**

2. **As you exhale, turn to your right and grasp the sides of the chair back with your hands.**

3. **As you inhale, bring your back and head up nice and tall; as you exhale, twist deeper.**

4. **Continue this sequence three times or until you reach your comfortable maximum and then stay for 4 to 6 breaths; repeat Steps 1 through 4 on the left side.**

Figure 18-10:
Seated sage twist.

Seated forward bend

These steps help you achieve this bend (illustrated in Figure 18-11).

1. **Start in the seated mountain posture.**

2. **As you exhale, bend forward from your hips and slide your hands forward and down your legs.**

3. **Let your head and arms hang down and relax in the folded position for 4 to 6 breaths.**

4. **For a nice ending, use the seated mountain posture. Close your eyes and choose focus breathing (Chapter 5) or a relaxation technique (Chapter 4) for two to five minutes.**

Figure 18-11:
Seated
forward bend.

Cherish the chair routine: Level II

This routine is more challenging than level I (see the preceding section) and should take about 15 to 20 minutes. (But don't let the word *challenging* scare you — our model Tony is well into his 80s!) Pick one of Chapter 5's Yoga breathing techniques and use it for the entire routine. The instructions and photos here show you how it's done.

 This routine also works in an office environment for any age group.

Seated mountain posture

Figure 18-12 illustrates this posture. Here's how it works:

1. **Sit comfortably in a chair with your back extended and your eyes either open or closed.**

2. **Hang your arms at your sides and visualize a vertical line down the middle of your ears, shoulders, hips, and the backs of your hands; stay for eight to ten breaths.**

Figure 18-12:
Seated mountain posture.

Seated mountain double arm variation I

1. **Start in the seated mountain posture (see the preceding section).**

2. **As you inhale, raise your arms from the front up and overhead.**

   Try to bring your arms alongside of your ears with your palms forward as in Figure 18-13, but don't force it.

3. **As you exhale, lower your arms back to your sides.**

4. **Repeat Steps 1 through 3 four to six times.**

Figure 18-13:
*Seated
mountain
double arm
variation I.*

Seated mountain double arm variation II

Figure 18-14 and the following steps show you how to achieve this pose.

1. **Start in the seated mountain posture.**

2. **As you inhale, raise your arms from the front, up and overhead.**

3. **Interlace your fingers and reverse your palms up toward the ceiling.**

4. **Keeping your arms soft, hold your arms alongside your ears for 4 to 6 breaths.**

Figure 18-14:
Seated mountain double arm variation II.

Seated triangle posture

Refer to Figure 18-15 for a visual of this posture and then follow these steps:

1. **Start in the seated mountain posture and, as you inhale, raise your right arm out and up from the right side with your palm rotated inward toward your head.**

2. **As you exhale, lean your right arm, head, and torso to the left as you drop your left arm down.**

   Keep your hips on the seat of the chair.

3. **Hold Step 2 for 4 to 6 breaths and then repeat Steps 1 through 3 on the opposite side (with the left arm).**

Figure 18-15:
Seated
triangle
posture.

Seated pigeon posture

Figure 18-16 demonstrates this posture; here's how you do it.

Don't try this posture if you've had a hip replacement.

1. **Start in the seated mountain posture.**

2. **As you exhale, bring your bent right knee directly up and then hold the outside of that knee with your right hand and the outside of your right heel with your left hand.**

3. **Place the outside of your right ankle on top of your left thigh just above your left knee; drop your right knee down towards the floor to a comfortable level.**

4. **Stay for 4 to 6 breaths and then repeat on the other side.**

You can slowly and gently move your top knee up and down a few times to limber the hip joint before you relax and breathe.

413

Figure 18-16:
Seated pigeon
posture.

Seated warrior I chair variation

Check out Figure 18-17 for the proper positioning on this posture and then follow these steps to complete it yourself:

1. **Straddle your chair sideways with the back of the chair on your right.**

2. **Keep your right knee bent in a right angle and try to straighten your back (left) leg with your toes or foot on the floor.**

3. **As you inhale, raise both arms forward and up until they're alongside your ears.**

4. **Stay in this position for 4 to 6 breaths and then repeat Steps 1 through 3 on the other (left) side, holding Step 3 for 4 to 6 breaths.**

Figure 18-17:
Seated warrior I chair variation.

Seated camel posture

The following steps and Figure 18-18 show you how to execute this posture:

1. **Start in the seated mountain posture.**

2. **Move to the front edge of your chair; reach back with your hands and hold the back of your seat or the sides of your chair back.**

3. **As you inhale, lengthen your head and neck up and then slowly look up at the ceiling; hold this position for 4 to 6 breaths.**

If you have neck problems, begin by just looking forward and then try looking up gradually over a period of time. If this head movement causes any pain or dizziness, leave it out.

Figure 18-18:
Seated camel posture.

Seated forward bend

These steps help you achieve this bend (illustrated in Figure 18-19).

1. **Start in the seated mountain posture.**

2. **As you exhale, bend forward from your hips and slide your hands forward and down your legs.**

3. **Let your head and arms hang down and relax in the folded position for 4 to 6 breaths.**

4. **Finish the sequence in the seated mountain posture. Close your eyes and use focus breathing (Chapter 5) or a relaxation technique (Chapter 4) for two to five minutes.**

Figure 18-19:
Seated
forward bend.

Chapter 19

Prop Art: The Why and How of Simple Props

The mainstay for any Yoga practice is, of course, the body-mind itself. However, props — physical means of support — may enhance your Yoga experience, especially if you're a beginner.

Traditionally, yogis and yoginis have relied on just a few basic props for their postural, breathing, and meditation practice — a bundle of grass or a tiger skin to sit on, a T-shaped arm rest (called *hamsa danda*) for prolonged meditation, and a *neti pot,* which looks like an undersized pitcher, for cleansing the nasal cavities with lukewarm (often salted) water prior to practicing breath control. Unfortunately, most Westerners' lifestyles and diets produce neither a naturally balanced mind nor a well-trained body, so a lot of these folks (especially beginners) often need to incorporate props into their Yoga to help encourage proper alignment.

That said, your own body is often all the prop you need. For example, the principle of *Forgiving Limbs* (which we cover in Chapter 3), in which you bend your knees and elbows, allows you to enjoy the function and benefits of a given posture even if your body isn't flexible enough to assume the posture's *classic* (traditionally taught) form. Many may benefit from the use of simple aids in addition to their bent limbs, so we discuss some of these external props in this chapter. When you use them intelligently, props can help you practice with pleasure in spite of tight hamstrings, stiff hips, and an inflexible back.

Of course, using props has both pros and cons, but this chapter gives you enough information to make your own decisions about what you want to include in your Yoga practice; throughout the book, we point out where you may benefit from using a prop in a posture and show you how to use it.

Examining the Pros and Cons of Props

As with anything in life, doing Yoga with props has its up-sides and downsides. The following sections list some of the benefits and disadvantages of using props, but you have to determine on your own how props can help support your Yoga practice.

Exploring the advantages of props

One of the great things about using props in your Yoga practice is that you can use them as extensively as you want or not at all. A folded blanket under your hips can make all the difference when you want to sit cross-legged for more than a couple of minutes, and a wall can be a welcome support for your legs or back while you're doing particular postures. Here are a few more prop plusses:

- They give you the added advantage of leverage in many postures.

- They help to improve your alignment, balance, and stability.

- Props like the Body Slant (which we discuss later in the chapter) provide the benefits of a classic inversion such as a headstand without compressing your neck.

- They allow you to participate more fully in a group class. With safe tools, you can perform some postures that would otherwise be inaccessible to you instead of hanging out in easier or resting postures until the group comes back to your level.

- They are, for the most part, relatively inexpensive and usually last for a long time.

Looking at props' drawbacks

Although Yoga props have their benefits, they do have some downsides as well. Keep the following in mind as you evaluate whether a prop is right for you:

- Given the advantage of a prop, some people go too far in a posture and injure themselves. Rather than try to look like a magazine-cover or Yoga-calendar model, listen to your own body's needs.

- You have to carry some props around with you when you go to a class.

- You can become too dependent on props, which inhibits your progress.

- Some props take time to set up and take down and can break the flow of a class.

- Some props are expensive.

Going Prop Hunting at Home

The human species prides itself on its use of tools, and Yoga's growing popularity in the Western world has spawned an industry of Yoga-related props — gear that can be complicated and costly. But useful props can be as simple as items lying around your house. Usually, a couple of blankets, a strap, a chair, or a wall for support is all that you need.

Yoga has always favored an experimental approach, and we suggest that you proceed in the same way. Find out for yourself what works for you and what doesn't. Instead of giving up on a challenging posture, experiment with one or the other recommended prop. For instance, if you can't sit comfortably with your legs folded in the tailor's seat *(sukhasana),* try placing a folded blanket or firm pillow under your hips. The following sections explain how common household finds can prop up your Yoga session.

Working with a wall

Walls are a great prop — they're everywhere, they're free, and best of all, they're versatile. You can use a wall in a great variety of postures: to support your buttocks and improve the angle of your forward bend, to brace your back heel in the standing postures, or to support the backs of your legs in the reclining raised-legs relaxation position.

Walls also can support you in the more advanced inverted postures, such as the half shoulder stand (see Chapter 10), or as a frame of reference by which you can check your posture and alignment.

Using a blanket for more than bedding

Besides the obvious use of keeping you warm during relaxation, blankets can prop your hips in sitting postures, your head and neck in lying postures, and your waist in prone back bends like the locust posture. You also can use blankets as protective padding under your knees when kneeling. The firmness of the blanket is important. You want something under your knees or neck that doesn't sink or collapse, as does a padded blanket or comforter. Always use a firm, flat blanket and be sure to fold it thickly (or use more than one) when you need to raise your hips (or head or shoulders).

 Most blankets nowadays are made out of synthetic materials (or a synthetic/wool blend) — a relief for people with wool allergies.

Choosing a chair for comfort

A folding metal chair or a sturdy wooden chair without arms can have multiple uses as a Yoga prop. Many (if not most) beginners have a hard time sitting on the floor for prolonged periods during meditation or breathing exercises, and sitting on a chair is a great alternative to sitting on the floor. Make sure, though, that your feet aren't dangling; if they don't easily touch the floor, place them on a phone book. Students with back problems often use a chair during the relaxation phase at the end of a Yoga class. Lying on your back and placing your lower legs up on a chair, combined

Prop proliferation

Yoga props and accessories from around the world are now big business in the United States. Yoga Master BKS Iyengar of Pune (pronounced *poon-ah*) more than any other teacher has influenced the development of props for Hatha Yoga in modern times. Americans, however, have made some of their own breakthroughs in the area of Yoga-inspired props.

Yoga teacher Larry Jacobs of Newport Beach, California, invented the Body Slant (which we describe later in "Turning to inversion props") and offers an entire line of safe and practical inversion furniture through mainstream mail-order catalogs nationally. Renowned sports medicine physician Leroy R. Perry, Jr., DC, in Los Angeles, California, has developed specialized inversion products, known as Dr. Perry's spinal decompressor devices, used by Yoga teachers and Yoga enthusiasts internationally.

with guided relaxation techniques from the instructor, can really help to release back tension or pain. You can find numerous books and magazine articles about doing your entire Yoga practice in a chair, with suggestions for ways to take Yoga chair breaks around the house or in your office for a quick pick-me-up.

Stretching with a strap

You most frequently use a strap with postures that involve stretching the hamstrings, most commonly from a supine reclining (lying on your back) or sitting position. Someone's old karate belt or necktie works great, but so does a rolled-up towel or a bathrobe belt. You also can order an "official" Yoga strap from one of the mail-order companies we list in the appendix.

Searching Out Props You May Want to Purchase

As you gain comfort and confidence with Yoga practice, you're sure to become curious about the array of props you either see being used in class or hear about from your association with fellow Yoga practitioners. Whether you plan to spend freely as you experiment with the best props for your personal situation, or you expect to approach buying a bit more conservatively, keep in mind that you're likely to find a sweeping range of merchandise and price tags out there in consumer land. By investing wisely — with product research, plus understanding your own needs — you can enjoy greater rewards from your Yoga experience. Figure 19-1 shows you walls, straps, bolsters, blocks, and chairs — all common Yoga props. The following sections give you more information on buying them; check out the preceding section for ways you can mimic some props with household items.

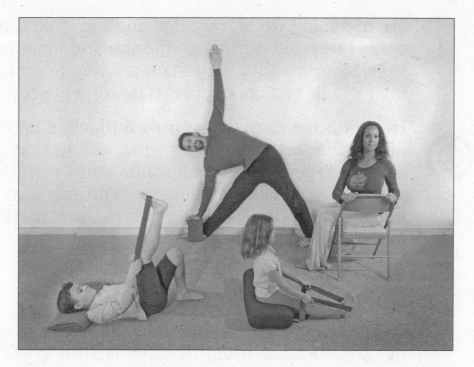

Figure 19-1: *Common Yoga props.*

Supporting alignment with the help of blocks

Some styles of Yoga incorporate blocks for improving or facilitating certain postures. You may find a block helpful in standing twists, when your bottom hand can't make it to the floor, or in standing forward bends, to support your hands. Two blocks are ideal, but you can get by with one. If you use a block, it should be firm. Some students prefer the more substantial feel and heft of a wooden block, or they may like the lightness of foam or other light materials (especially if they drop the block on a floor or foot). For beginners, put the block down on the floor horizontally or lying flat. Think of the block as a raised floor to support you. Try not to clutch the block with your hands — just use it to aid your balance.

Commercially, blocks are available in a variety of materials, including wood, recycled and new foam, bamboo, and cork. The price varies with the size and material and ranges from $8 up to $30, with foam tending to be less expensive than wood, and cork somewhere in between.

If you decide to make your own block, a good standard is nine inches high, six inches wide, and four inches deep. Be sure that the block is well-sanded and varnished to eliminate the possibility of splinters. You can also tightly wrap up an old hardback book or two in some masking tape and use that for support.

Bolstering support with pillows

Bolsters are large, firm, usually rectangular or cylindrical pillows. You use them to support your knees in reclining postures, to help release your lower back and to raise your buttocks in forward bends, and to help soften tight hips and hamstrings. You can also place bolsters under your upper back to help open your chest when you lie over them. During the stress of pregnancy, bolsters are a great support for the side-lying posture (see Chapter 16). A good standard size for bolsters is 6 x 12 x 25 inches for the rectangular bolsters and 9 x 27 inches for the cylindrical shape.

Bolsters are usually made of thick cotton batting with a removable canvas covering that you can wash, and they come in a range of sizes, materials, and prices. Expect to pay somewhere in the range of $35 to $70, depending upon your taste and needs. You can also buy a pranayama bolster (see Chapter 5) that is long and thin (about 8 x 30 inches). One bolster is usually plenty for your personal use.

You can create your own bolsters by using thickly rolled blankets. In a pinch, sofa or bed pillows work, too — if they're not too soft.

Eyeing the many applications of eye bags

Eye bags, also called *eye pillows,* are small bags filled with light materials (usually plastic pellets) that yogis and yoginis use for various relaxation techniques. Although an eye bag may seem self-explanatory, there's actually more to eye bags than meets the, well, eye. They of course block light and other visual stimuli, which helps quiet the brain; they also put gentle pressure on your eyes, which slows your heart rate. You can just cover your eyes with a towel, but the effect isn't quite the same.

Eye bags are available in many shapes and sizes. Some eye bags are packed with herbal essences, which adds the incentive (in-scent-ive?) of aroma therapy, but be sure the perfume isn't so strong it becomes bothersome. Eye bags are usually about 4 x 8 inches and cost from $10 to $20, depending on which type you choose; some more-expensive models tie down like a mask, which is usually unnecessary. (Check out the appendix for more on locating props.) You usually place one eye bag across the top of both eyes while you're in a lying position on your back.

 If you decide to make your own eye bags, use materials such as cotton stuffed with rice, or silk stuffed with flaxseed. Even stuffing an old sock does the job. Be sure to do a good job on the seams — you don't want flaxseed in your eyes!

Turning to inversion props

We purposely omitted the headstand and the full shoulder stand from this book because we feel that these postures require the guidance of a competent Yoga teacher. Because Western-world necks have become so weak and vulnerable, many physicians and a large number of chiropractors, orthopedists, and osteopaths aren't in favor of inverted Yoga postures such as the headstand, the full shoulder stand, and the plow because they can compress the neck. Because the benefits of inversion and reversing the pull of gravity are so great (as we cover in Chapter 10), many entrepreneurs have attempted to create safe and effective inversion devices.

You can now find quite a selection of inversion apparatuses to suit various bodies and budgets. One that we like for its effectiveness, safety, and convenience is the Body Slant created by yogi Larry Jacobs and shown in Figure 19-2. It's the high-tech version of what used to be called Grandma's Slant Board. These three pieces of firm foam that fold and unfold easily make inversion safe and simple. Just lie back for 10 minutes to receive the rejuvenating effects of inversion.

Figure 19-2:
The Body Slant is safe and effective.

 Ask your physician before using any new exercise device to be sure that the prop is right for your personal situation.

 Avoid using the Body Slant or any other inversion prop if you have the following conditions: glaucoma or *retinopathy* (disease of the retina), hiatal hernia, high blood pressure, heart disease, or a past stroke.

Part IV

Yoga as a Lifestyle

The 5th Wave   By Rich Tennant

"I convinced him to practice Yoga at work. He's more calm, focused, and I keep all the change that falls out of his pocket."

In this part . . .

In this part, we take a two-pronged approach. We start by introducing you to the ways in which Yoga is so much more than physical exercise. We show you how you can adopt Yoga as a lifestyle that brings you inner peace and happiness, as well as the capacity to become a beacon of light for your family, friends, coworkers, and others. We talk about your enormous spiritual and the power of living with moral integrity.

Then, we show you how you can maintain your lifestyle by making Yoga part of your life even when your aches and pains are getting you down. We provide examples of specific yogic exercises known to be safe and helpful, and a five-step plan to prevent back problems from becoming chronic. We also discuss how to know when using Yoga therapeutically on your own is safe, how to seek out a Yoga therapist, and when you should consult a doctor.

Chapter 20

Yoga Throughout the Day

• •

In This Chapter

▶ Applying Yoga throughout the day
▶ Looking inward for health and harmony
▶ Developing moral practices
▶ Reaping rewards from self-discipline

• •

The postures and breathing exercises of Hatha Yoga — some of which we cover in preceding chapters — are merely a couple of tools from Yoga's well-stocked storehouse. When you practice them correctly, they're extremely useful and potent in helping you regain or maintain your physical and mental health. Practicing postures and breathing can stabilize and boost your body's vitality and even harmonize your emotions and strengthen your mind.

But postures and breathing exercises are only a beginning; they're only two steps in the eightfold path of Raja Yoga (see Chapter 1 for more about Raja Yoga and the eightfold path). The real power of Yoga is unlocked when you approach it as a lifestyle or spiritual path. Yoga is a conscious

431

way of life; it contains everything you need in order to transform your entire day. Just as a grand piano allows you to play music in eight octaves, Yoga gives you the means to tap into your full potential as a human being.

In this chapter, we show you how you can connect with your deeper potential and live your entire day the Yoga way. This approach includes paying proper attention to moral values, which are an important aspect of all branches and schools of Yoga but are often overlooked by Western practitioners.

Living Your Day the Yoga Way

When you decide to pursue Yoga as a lifestyle or spiritual discipline, you must be willing to practice it 24 hours a day, 7 days a week. You may think that this total commitment sounds difficult, and with good reason — living this way is truly a challenge! At least, staying on track is difficult while you're busy creating new habit patterns by laying down new pathways in your brain. After you change your thoughts and behavior, living the Yoga way is as easy as living any other routine, except the yogic lifestyle is far from routine.

Turning your face toward a Yoga morning

For thousands of years, Yoga practitioners have begun the day at sunrise, a time considered to be favorable and especially potent for meditation, prayer, and tapping into your highest potential. Called *brahma-muhurta* in Sanskrit (*brahmah moo-hoor-tah,* which means "hour of brahman," with brahman being the ultimate Reality), this time sets the right tone for the entire day.

Sunrise isn't only a quiet, peaceful time but also a time charged with symbolic significance for Yoga practitioners. Traditionally, the sun is celebrated as the first teacher, or *guru,* who brought the teachings of Yoga to humanity. According to Yoga, the sun is a symbol for the spirit, which shines with undiminished brightness forever. The sun salutation exercise described in Chapter 13 is one way yogis acknowledge their reverence for the inner sun.

Of course, India (Yoga's native home) is blessed with a lot of sunshine. Even if your climate doesn't offer much physical sun, you can still enjoy sunrise as a special, daily occasion — just ponder the sun's profound symbolism!

Here are some suggestions for transforming an otherwise mundane daily routine into a meaningful ritual that can energize and prepare you for the onslaught of the day:

- **Create a peaceful mood in your heart and remember your connection with everyone and everything.** Do this work as soon as you wake up and before opening your eyes and getting out of bed. If you believe in a divine being (call it God, Goddess, or higher Self), this moment is good for inwardly aligning yourself to it/him/her.

- **Write down any significant dreams.** When you live an active life of self-transformation, dreams often carry important messages. They may mirror and confirm your present inner development or stream of experiences, or they may provide you with a key for understanding what you're going through. If you don't write down your dreams shortly after waking, you're likely to forget them. If you find that they fade from your mind rapidly, you may want to consider jotting them down in a diary before making your daily resolution (*samkalpa,* pronounced *sahm-kahl-pah*), which we cover next.

✔ **Affirm your highest resolve.** For example, repeat (aloud or in your mind) your resolution, such as "I intend to act all day long in accordance to the highest spiritual and moral principles," "I intend to be (more) compassionate today," "I intend to harm no one and benefit as many people as possible," "I intend to think only positive, benign thoughts today," and so on. Repeat your intention *(samkalpa)* with great conviction three or more times.

Remembering an affirmation throughout the day is often difficult for beginning students. Try carrying something small around with you, such as a pebble, a button, or a ring, that can jog your memory whenever you see or touch it.

✔ **Before getting out of bed, consciously relax and take ten deep breaths.**

✔ **Stretch and thus fire up your muscles while you're still in bed.**

✔ **Use the bathroom, wash, and brush your teeth.**

✔ **Meditate.** If you meditate sitting on your bed,

your mind inevitably associates "bed" with "sleep." See Chapter 21 for more information on the art of meditation. Some authorities recommend that you do postures and breathing exercises before meditation, but we feel this preparation is only necessary when your mind tends to be sluggish in the early morning and you need to jump-start it. If you wake up easily and happily in the morning, use that time for meditation or prayer.

✔ **Do your Hatha Yoga program to vitalize your body and fortify your mind.**

If you can't practice in the morning (because, for example, you have to be at work when the rooster crows), make sure that you leave room in your schedule for Hatha Yoga and/or meditation at some other time during the day or in the evening. Even a few minutes of postures and breathing exercises are better than no exercises at all. But more importantly, always start your day right by making your resolution upon waking and centering yourself by breathing consciously.

 If you have a family, make formal agreements with your partner and/or children so that you can practice Yoga as undisturbed as possible. Be sure that everyone is aware of and honors your private time. If need be, lock your door or post a reminder sign. You may not always be able to get private time, especially when you have young children. In that case, try to do whatever practices you can while you're still in bed, and then include your children in your Yoga program. As a parent, you're the best role model for your children, and even toddlers can participate in your Yoga practice.

Some people are super-busy — going to bed late at night after they're exhausted and starting out the next morning

Yoga with your youngsters

If you have young children and have no leisure time to practice Yoga on your own, don't despair! Make the most of the situation. As the saying goes, if you can't beat them, join them. Your kids will love it — at least while the novelty lasts. Depending on their age and general disposition, the youngsters may get used to this little routine and happily participate in it or, if not, they may at least allow you to practice your own Yoga routine without too many interruptions. If you don't want them to get bored, you must make the session fun for the kids. As you well know, the universe revolves around children and their needs — until they learn otherwise. Your own peacefulness can definitely have a calming effect on them. Check out Chapter 17 for more on doing Yoga with kids.

still feeling tired. A regular Hatha Yoga routine can give you energy, making regular practice well worth the time it takes. Beyond the physical and mental benefits, Yoga provides much-needed quiet time, where you can be by yourself without distraction. If your situation permits, arrange to have 15 minutes a day that you can consider all yours. Make a creative deal with your partner and/or children that can benefit everyone.

Or, if you live alone and feel the pressures of time and attention to lots of details, just negotiate an agreement with the person who shows up in your mirror. You can be a better friend to that face if you set aside some time for inward glances.

Practicing Yoga throughout the day

You have many opportunities to apply the wisdom of Yoga

as activities and situations during the day. Whether you stay at home with your children or hold down a job outside the home, you have at your disposal an array of tools from Yoga's versatile toolbox for all circumstances. Here are only a few situations in which you can fruitfully apply yogic wisdom (although any situation can benefit from good Yoga practice):

- Encountering heavy traffic during your daily commute to and from work

- Dealing with customers, a demanding boss, or fellow employees

- Enjoying breakfast, lunch, and dinner (see the nearby sidebar "The yogic art of conscious eating")

- Experiencing pregnancy and childbirth (head to Chapter 16)

- Responding when your child's behavior leaves much to be desired

- Living through a health crisis

- Enjoying vacations and holidays

- Doing the daily shopping

- Grieving over the death of a loved one

- Watching television

- Having sex

To all these situations you can bring awareness, which is the foundation for all other positive attitudes and practices. You can also bring understanding, patience, calmness, forgiveness, kindness, compassion, love, good humor, and a host of other virtues. By practicing various Yoga techniques, you can also calm your mind and raise your energy level or bring energy to others.

Don't think of the world as "out there" and your Yoga practice as "in here." Because Yoga connects inside and outside, such a distinction is artificial. Allow your practice to flow over into all situations. You're never so busy that you can't transform a few seconds of free time into meaningful time through Yoga: Exhale deeply, center yourself, silently recite a *mantra,* or bless someone.

Incorporating Yoga into nighttime routines

When you live Yoga as a spiritual discipline, the practice extends even to your sleep. In Chapter 4, we give you a relaxation technique that's better than any sleeping pill for preparing you for sleep. You can make this technique even more powerful by repeating the same intention *(samkalpa)* that you also use upon waking; flip to "Turning your face toward a Yoga morning" earlier in the chapter for more on the samkalpa. Repeat your intention when your relaxation is deepest and before emerging from it or falling asleep.

The yogic art of conscious eating

What you eat forms your body. In turn, the condition of your body and especially the nervous system affects your mind, which affects your entire life. Thus the traditional maxim "You are what you eat" holds true to a certain degree. Yoga masters have typically been vegetarians, favoring grains, legumes, and fruit. In your diet, stick as close to Mother Nature as possible.

As important as what you eat is how you eat. Of all the recommendations made by Yoga masters, the single most important is to *practice moderation*. This habit is called *mitahara* (from *mita* or

---

438

"moderate" and *ahara* or "food" in Sanskrit, pronounced *mee-tah-hah-rah*). Basically, you avoid both overeating and starving yourself.

Overeating not only puts pounds on you but also multiplies toxins in your body and makes you feel emotionally weighed down. Similarly, if you don't feed your body adequately, you weaken it and also risk causing disease. The best policy is to eat only when you're hungry (not just peckish). The right amount to eat varies from person to person and also according to climate and season. Find out for yourself by trial and error. Remember, though, that certain health conditions require frequent eating.

Another important yogic rule about diet is to eat with awareness. Here are some simple suggestions for changing unyogic or mechanical habits while you eat:

- ✔ Calm down first if you're agitated.

- ✔ Keep your attention on the task of eating.

- ✔ Eat slowly and chew your food well.

- ✔ Pay attention to the wonderful taste sensations in your mouth.

- ✔ Breathe.

- ✔ Be grateful for your food.

Sleeping peacefully with lucid dreaming

You can benefit from taking note of your dreams, keeping a diary of at least the more significant ones. But dedicated yogis and yoginis seek to transform their dream life altogether by training themselves in *lucid dreaming,* a special state of consciousness in which you retain a degree of self-

439

awareness while dreaming. In other words, you know that you're dreaming and, with practice, even are able to direct your dreams. Usually lucid dreaming occurs spontaneously, but by priming your mind before going to sleep you can increase the likelihood of becoming self-aware in the midst of a dream. If you're interested in exploring this art, we recommend that you study the resources listed in this book's appendix. In the meantime, here are some pointers for programming yourself to dream lucidly:

✔ Become generally more aware of your thoughts, feelings, and sensations.

✔ Take an interest in your dreams.

✔ Get up a couple of hours earlier than usual and go about your regular chores.

✔ Slip back into bed and think about lucid dreaming and what sort of dream you want to create for about 30 minutes.

✔ Allow yourself at least two hours for dreaming before finally getting up.

✔ Induce lucid dreaming by doing the kind of deep relaxation exercise (Yoga Nidra) that we describe in Chapter 4.

✔ Clearly form the intention to dream lucidly.

You may not succeed the first or second time you try, but then again, pleasant surprises may be just a dream away!

Aiming toward awareness through lucid waking

More important than lucid dreaming is *lucid waking* — the

440

art of being present in the moment, of living with mindfulness throughout the day. In a way, lucid dreaming is an extension of lucid waking. If you acquire the knack of becoming aware in the dream state but continue to sleepwalk in your waking life, you can't expect to gain very much. If you're aware but lacking in understanding or wisdom in the waking state, you also lack understanding or wisdom in the dream state. Yoga is first and foremost about lucid waking, which means penetrating the illusions and delusions of ordinary life with the searchlight of full awareness. After you clear your mind of its inherent misconceptions and biases, you can bring the same clear mind to unordinary states of consciousness, including dreaming and deep sleep.

Approaching mindfulness in deep sleep

For the serious Yoga practitioner, even deep sleep isn't a no-man's land. On the contrary, dreamless sleep is a great opportunity for breaking into higher levels of consciousness. After you're able to retain mindful awareness during the dream state, you can extend your awareness to those periods where the mind is devoid of contents. The great Yoga masters are continuously aware throughout the day and the night. They're never unconscious, because they have realized the spirit or Self, which is pure consciousness.

If constant awareness sounds exhausting, consider the deep peacefulness that the Yoga masters are able to achieve. Pure consciousness is the simplest thing in the world. Hence, it's called the *natural state,* or *sahaja-avastha (sah-hah-jah ah-vahst-hah).* By comparison, the mind is vastly complicated. Just remember how thinking (especially when you're obsessing over something) can be incredibly exhausting.

441

Swami Rama baffles scientists

In 1969, Swami Rama volunteered to have his yogic abilities tested at the Menninger Foundation in Topeka, Kansas. Among other things, he demonstrated his ability to produce all types of brain waves at will. He remained fully aware even when producing the slow delta waves characteristic of deep sleep. In fact, he was able to remember what happened during his supposed deep sleep much better than did the researchers themselves. Two years later, Swami Rama founded the Himalayan Institute in Honesdale, Pennsylvania, which continues to spread his teachings. Check out the appendix for the Institute's address.

Seeking Your Higher Self by Discovering the True You

However they may conceive the ultimate goal, all schools of Yoga seek to open a door to your true nature, which we call the *spirit* or *higher Self.* You can find as many approaches to Self-realization (or enlightenment) as you can human beings. Everyone's spiritual journey is unique, yet everyone's inner evolution follows certain universal principles. That fundamental process is marked by progressive *self-observation, self-understanding, self-discipline,* and *self-transcendence,* which are all interconnected practices. The most significant principle is that in order to discover your essential nature, you must overcome the gravity pull of your ordinary habit patterns (laid down as neural pathways in your brain).

Observing yourself

In Yoga, you simply begin to observe yourself. Staying in tune with yourself is different from the neurotic self-watching that's merely a form of self-involvement. *Self-observation* means being consciously aware of how you think and behave without judging yourself in any way.

Self-observation includes noticing — in a nonjudgmental way — how you react to people and situations. For instance, you may discover that in many ways, you're often overly critical or too gullible and accommodating. Or you may determine that you tend to be rather inward and afraid of engaging life or that you never think before you leap. The natural calmness that you create through Yoga's physical exercises can help you start uncovering your tendencies — without collapsing into self-recrimination or exploding into anger with others.

Understanding yourself

Based on self-observation, self-understanding involves grasping the deeper reasons for your habit patterns. Ultimately, *self-understanding* is the realization that all your thoughts and behaviors revolve around the ego, an artificial psychological pole. Your ego allows you to identify yourself in a very specific way. For example:

"I'm Frank, a 35-year-old, Caucasian male and a United States citizen. I'm 5 foot 11 inches tall, have an athletic build, weigh 165 pounds, and have blue eyes and brown hair. I'm married, have two children, and am an electronic engineer who likes to go parachuting. I'm a capitalist, reasonably ambitious, but not very religious."

These ego-identifications are useful in your daily life — as long as they don't cause you to feel separated from your spiritual core or to create barriers to other people.

You have to be very careful not to take the ego habit too seriously; the ego is nothing more than a way of quickly identifying yourself both verbally and psychologically. It's not your true nature, the spirit or Self. Most importantly, it's not an actual entity in its own right but merely something you habitually do. The ego is based on the process of self-contraction *(atma-samkoca,* pronounced *aht-mah sahm-koh-chah).* The symbol for the ego is a clenched fist. Yoga shows you how to release that fist and engage life from the viewpoint of the spirit or Self, which is in harmonious relationship with everyone and everything.

Practicing self-discipline

When a seed sprouts, it must first push through the soil before it can benefit from the sunlight. Similarly, before you can experience the higher levels of Yoga, you must overcome the built-in lethargy of your ego-driven personality, which doesn't want to change. Self-observation and self-understanding become increasingly effective through the practice of *self-discipline* — the steady cultivation of spiritual practices.

By exercising voluntary self-control over your thoughts, behaviors, and energies, you can gradually transform your body-mind into a finely tuned instrument for higher spiritual realizations and harmonious living. You can't practice self-discipline without frustrating the ego a little, because the ego always tends to move along the path of least resistance. Yogic practice creates the necessary resistance to spark further growth in you.

Transcending yourself

Self-transcendence is at the heart of the spiritual process. This impulse and practice of going beyond the ego-contraction in every moment — through self-observation, self-understanding, and self-discipline — comes to full blossom in the great event of enlightenment, when your entire being is transformed by the spirit, or Self (see Chapter 21).

Making Inroads into the Eightfold Path with Moral Discipline

The eightfold path of Yoga, as we outline it in Chapter 1, is a useful model for the stages of the yogic process. In the following sections, we explain the first limb of the eightfold path in more detail because along with the second limb, it gives you the essential moral foundation for practicing Yoga successfully. We start with the five practices of moral discipline *(yama),* which Yoga insists that you must practice under all circumstances. They're the same moral virtues that you find in all the world's great religious traditions:

- Nonharming or *ahimsa* (pronounced *ah-heem-sah*)

- Truthfulness or *satya* (pronounced *saht-yah*)

- Nonstealing or *asteya* (pronounced *ahs-the-yah*)

- Chastity or *brahmacarya* (pronounced *brah-mah-chahr-yah*)

- Greedlessness or *aparigraha* (pronounced *ah-pah-ree-grah-hah*)

These five disciplines are meant to harmonize your interpersonal life and are especially important in today's enormously complex world. Much of the social chaos in today's world is due to the collapse of a common system of basic moral values. Yoga reminds you that you can't attain self-fulfillment in isolation from others. You can't hope to realize your higher nature without fostering what's good and beautiful in your day-to-day life in interaction with your family, friends, co-workers, teachers, and students. Thus, universally recognized moral virtues are the rich soil in which you plant all your other efforts on the path of inner growth and ultimate Self-realization (or enlightenment).

Yoga understands these virtues to be all-comprehensive, extending not only to your actions but also to your language and even your thoughts. In other words, you're called to abstain from doing wrong to others, speaking wrong of them, as well as poisoning them with your thoughts.

Vowing to do no harm

The practice of nonharming comes — or should come — into play hundreds of times a day. The more sensitive you become toward the effect you have on others, the more you're called to live with moral mindfulness. How do you practice the virtue of nonharming in your life? You may think of yourself as a fairly harmless individual because you don't physically or verbally abuse anyone, but have you ever started or listened to gossip? And what about feeling negatively toward an annoying client or customer or an inconsiderate driver who just took your parking space?

Nonharming is not only abstaining from harmful actions, speech, and thoughts but also actively doing what's appropriate in a given moment to avoid unnecessary pain to others. For example, even withholding a smile or kind word from someone when you sense that the gesture may benefit that person is a form of harming.

446

In order to live, humans involuntarily harm and even kill other beings — just think of the billions of microorganisms in your food and even in your own body that give up their lives so that you can stay alive and be healthy. The ideal of nonharming is just that: an ideal to which you may aspire. The concept calls for abstaining from deliberately harming other beings. As a useful exercise, ask yourself these questions:

- How many times today have I spoken harshly?

- When did I last kill a harmless spider instead of leaving it alone or relocating it?

- Are my thoughts about things and people predominantly pessimistic, overly optimistic, or simply realistic?

- When I have to correct someone's behavior, do I merely criticize or also encourage?

Yoga definitely expects you to control your anger and murderous thoughts — not to be confused with merely suppressing your feelings (which never works anyway). Yoga also encourages you to cultivate, step by step, better habits and mental dispositions. As you become more peaceful and content, you don't react so strongly and irrationally to life's pressures but rather become more and more able to go with the flow — with awareness, a smile, and a helping hand. According to Yoga, a person grounded in nonharming is surrounded by such an aura of peace that even wild beasts become tame.

If you become aware of the various ways in which you harm others through your thoughts, words, and actions, don't succumb to feeling overwhelmed with guilt. That negative response is just another way of perpetuating violence. Simply acknowledge the situation, feel remorse, resolve to behave differently, and then also actively change your mental, verbal, and physical behavior.

Telling the truth all the time

These days, many folks seem to believe that truth is relative. Yoga, however, insists that facts and perspectives are many but truth is always one and that truthfulness *(satya)* is a supreme moral virtue. Truth is the cement that holds together good relationships and entire societies.

The sorry condition of modern society says something about the society's commitment (or lack thereof) to truth. For instance, consider the following questions:

- ✔ Have you ever told a little white lie not because you wanted to protect someone but because you deemed it more convenient than to tell the truth?

- ✔ Have you ever prettified or omitted certain facts from your resumé to look more suitable to a prospective employer?

- ✔ Have you ever failed to declare taxable income (even that negligible amount that no one could possibly care about)?

- ✔ Have you ever instructed your spouse to say you aren't at home when an unwanted caller is on the phone for you?

- ✔ Have you ever lied about your age?

- ✔ Do you ever fail to keep your promises? (This question is a must for politicians.)

Probably, few people can answer all these questions with a resounding "No," unless, of course, they're lying to themselves. Admittedly, lies appear to vary by degree of severity. You may consider these examples fairly insignificant, and from a conventional point of view, they are. But Yoga doesn't let you off the hook so easily. Yogic practice values simplicity and clarity, whereas lying usually ends up being more complicated and confusing. Yoga is also concerned about the pathways you build in your brain. If you become accustomed to not telling the truth in little matters, sooner or later you may not be able to distinguish truth from falsehood in big matters as well.

Truthfulness is a marvelous tool for keeping your energy pure and your will undiluted. Of course, in your attempts to be truthful, you must bear the principal moral virtue of nonharming (covered in the preceding section) in mind. Life isn't black and white; many gray areas exist. If speaking the truth may bring more harm than good to another person, you're wise to remain silent. As with nonharming, your intention is the key.

Stealing means more than material theft

Nonstealing *(asteya),* the third moral discipline, is trickier than it looks at a casual glance. You need not be a pickpocket, shoplifter, bank robber, or embezzler to violate this virtue. From the perspective of Yoga, depriving someone of his or her due reward or good name is also theft. So is appropriating someone's ideas without due acknowledgment, stealing someone's boyfriend or girlfriend, or denying your child proper parental guidance.

To ponder the ideal of nonstealing, you may want to answer these questions:

- ✔ What percentage of your income do you allocate for charitable causes?

- Have you ever used someone else's time left on a parking meter, knowing that this widespread practice is actually against the law?

- Are any of your computer programs bootlegged copies (a criminal offense)?

- Did you ever withhold love from a family member or friend because you wanted to punish him or her?

Traditionally, those people who are well established in the virtue of nonstealing are described as always being sustained by life; they never lack anything for their further growth. The greatest antidote to the vice of stealing is generosity. A fulfilling life is a life that elegantly balances giving and taking.

Highly competitive Western society is designed to promote self-centeredness to the point where people constantly infringe the virtues of nonharming, truthfulness, and nonstealing. (Head to the preceding two sections for more on those first two values.) The kind of aggressive competitiveness rampant in the business world is all about elbowing your way to the top, beating the other guy, using any means necessary to outsmart your opponent, and winning the game at all costs.

Observing chastity in thought and deed

Chastity *(brahmacarya,* pronounced *brah-mah-chahr-yah),* which is a highly valued virtue in all traditional societies, means abstention from inappropriate sexual behavior. According to Yoga, only adults who are in a committed marriage or partnership should be sexually active; all others should practice sexual abstinence. For many Westerners, this standard is very difficult.

Yogically speaking, you must extend the ideal of chastity to action, speech, and even thought. We leave it up to you to determine where, in your own case, you can change your behavior to bring it more in line with Yoga's moral orientation. Bear in mind that Yoga isn't asking you to go against human nature, which includes sexuality. Rather, Yoga invites you to consider your higher spiritual potential. The Yoga masters recommend chastity not for prudish reasons but because it's an effective way of harnessing your body's vital energy. The practitioner who is firmly grounded in chastity supposedly obtains vigor or vitality.

 If you engage Yoga as a lifestyle or spiritual discipline, periodically taking stock of your virtues and vices can help you build toward achievement of your higher Self. When considering your sexuality, ask yourself these questions:

- Do I tend to use sexually suggestive or explicit language?

- Do I use sex for emotional security or for personal power?

- Am I flirtatious and, if so, why?

- Do I know the distinction between sex and love?

- Am I capable of true intimacy, or do I treat my partner as a sex object?

Acquiring more by living with less

Greed is a vice that underlies much of modern consumerism. From a yogic point of view, greed is a failed search for happiness, because whatever possessions you may acquire can't fulfill you. On the contrary, the more you're surrounded by "stuff," the more likely you are to experience a big gaping hole in your soul. Intrinsically, money and

451

possessions aren't "wrong," but few people ever master the art of relating to them properly. Instead of owning things, they're owned (controlled) by them.

Yoga holds high the ideal of voluntary simplicity — the choice to live simply. How do you measure up to it? Try to answer these questions honestly:

- Have you ever been called a miser?

- Do you have too much "stuff"?

- Do you expect to be pampered?

- Do you tend to overeat?

- Do you accumulate money and possessions because you worry about the future?

- Are you overly attached to your partner or child?

- Do you like to be the center of attention?

- Are you envious of your neighbors?

Yoga encourages you to cultivate the virtue of greedlessness in all matters. The Sanskrit word for this value is *aparigraha* (pronounced *ah-pah-ree-grah-ha*), which means "not grasping all round." The Yoga practitioner who is well-trained in the art of greedlessness is said to understand the deeper reason for his or her life. Behind this traditional wisdom lies a profound experience: As you loosen your grip on material possessions, you also let go of the ego, which is doing the gripping or grasping. As the ego-contraction relaxes, you increasingly become in touch with the abiding happiness of your true self. Then you realize that you need nothing at all to be happy. You're unconcerned about the future and live fully in the present. You aren't afraid to give freely to others and also share with them your inner abundance.

Adding other moral practices

In addition to the five moral virtues listed by Yoga master Patanjali in his *Yoga-Sutra,* other Yoga texts mention the following as belonging to the first limb of the eightfold path:

- Sympathy or *daya* (pronounced *dah-yah*)

- Compassion or *karuna* (pronounced *kah-roo-nah*)

- Integrity or *arjava* (pronounced *ahr-jah-vah*)

- Patience or *kshama* (pronounced *kshah-mah*)

- Steadfastness or *dhriti* (pronounced *dhree-tee*)

- Nonattachment or *vairagya* (pronounced *vie-rah-gyah*)

- Modesty or *hri* (pronounced *hree* — the initial letter *h* is sounded out loud)

- Humility or *amanitva* (pronounced *ah-mah-neet-vah*)

As you can see, Yoga has the highest expectations for a serious practitioner. But becoming a saint isn't the goal. Yoga is about freedom and happiness. The moral virtues are natural side effects of a life dedicated to Self-realization, or spiritual enlightenment (which we discuss in Chapter 21).

Exercising Yogic Self-Discipline

The second category or limb of the eightfold path is known as restraint *(niyama),* also translated as "self-restraint." We explain the second limb here because it's an integral part of the moral orientation of Yoga, which Western practitioners frequently give short shrift. According to Patanjali, restraint comprises five practices:

- ✔ Purity or *shauca* (pronounced *shau-chah* — the *au* sounds similar to *ow* in *cow*)

- ✔ Contentment or *samtosha* (pronounced *sahm-toh-shah*)

- ✔ Austerity or *tapas* (pronounced *tah-pahs*)

- ✔ Study or *svadhyaya* (pronounced *svahd-hyah-yah*)

- ✔ Dedication to a higher principle or *ishvara-pranidhana* (pronounced *eesh-vah-rah prah-need-hah-nah*)

Purifying mind and body

An old saying from the Puritan tradition suggests, "Cleanliness is next to godliness." Yoga goes further, stating that perfect purity and divinity are one and the same. All of Yoga is a process of self-purification. It begins with mental purification (through the practice of the moral disciplines described earlier in this chapter), proceeds to bodily cleansing (through various purification techniques, including postures and breath control), followed by more profound mental purification (through sensory inhibition, concentration, meditation, and the ecstatic state), and ends with realizing the perfect purity of the spirit itself.

The Sanskrit word for "purity" is *shauca,* which has the root meaning of "being radiant." The ultimate reality, or spirit, is pure radiance. As you clean the windows of your body-mind, you invite in more of the spirit's light. Accomplished Yoga masters have a radiance about them.

Calming the quest through contentment

Contentment *(samtosha)* is traditionally defined as being satisfied with what life presents to you. When you're content, you have joy in your heart and you don't need anything else. You can face life with great calm. That doesn't mean, however, that you need to avoid improvements in your situation, such as finding a better job or studying for a diploma or degree. It just means your quest for improvement doesn't come from a place of neediness or gnawing dissatisfaction.

Focusing with austerity

Austerity *(tapas)* entails all kinds of practices designed to test your willpower and awaken the energy locked away in your body. Traditionally, these tests included strict dieting or prolonged fasting, staying awake for several days, or sitting completely still in meditation directly under the hot Indian sun. Few of these practices are possible for modern Westerners, but the basic principle behind *tapas* (literally meaning "heat") is as valid now as it was thousands of years ago: Whenever you want to make progress on the path of Yoga, you must avoid wasting your energy on things that are irrelevant to your inner development. By carefully regulating your mental and physical behavior, you generate more energy for yogic practice.

But progress calls for overcoming all kinds of inner resistances. *Tapas* makes a demand on you, which creates a certain amount of inner heat. Change is never easy, and for many people, self-discipline is a big stumbling block. They tend to give up too soon. Yet self-discipline — through the strength of your will — is within reach. Just persist and observe how your goals move closer. For instance, your effort to overcome laziness and practice Yoga regularly is a form of *tapas,* which gradually strengthens your willpower.

A good way to practice *tapas* is by periodically going on a retreat, where you have nothing to distract you from your inner work. Retreats provide an opportunity to clearly see all your tendencies in technicolor and start turning them around by creating better patterns of thought and behavior. Austerity isn't about self-chastisement; it's an intelligent way of testing and strengthening your willpower. Remember, Yoga doesn't seek to increase pain and suffering but to remove it. Always be kind to yourself and, as your commitment to inner growth increases, don't hesitate to challenge yourself firmly.

Partnering research with self-study

Self-study *(svadhyaya)* is an important part of traditional Yoga, although contemporary Western practitioners who fail to understand its great value often neglect it. *Self-study* means both studying for yourself and studying yourself. Traditionally, this commitment involved poring over the sacred scriptures, reciting them, and meditating on their meanings. In this way, practitioners stayed in touch with the tradition and also gained self-understanding, because study of the scriptures always confronts you with yourself. For basic study, we recommend the following Yoga texts, which are all available in good English translations; flip to Chapter 1 for more on the specific branches of Yoga:

- ✔ *Yoga-Sutra* of Patanjali, the standard text on Raja Yoga

- ✔ *Bhagavad-Gita,* the earliest available Sanskrit text on Jnana Yoga, Karma Yoga, and Bhakti Yoga

- *Hatha-Yoga-Pradipika,* one of the classical manuals of Hatha Yoga

- *Yoga-Vasishtha,* a marvelous work on Jnana Yoga; filled with traditional stories and beautiful poetic imagery

- *Bhakti-Sutra* of Narada, a classical work on Bhakti Yoga

You can find full or partial translations of numerous Yoga texts in my (Georg's) *The Yoga Tradition* (Hohm Press). You can find more information in the appendix.

Why study the Yoga scriptures? They're the distillations of several thousand years of experimentation and experience. If you're serious about Yoga, why not benefit from the wisdom of the accomplished adepts of this tradition?

Today, you can usefully extend your study to include not only important Yoga scriptures but also contemporary knowledge that can further your self-understanding. Yoga practitioners who recognize the great ideas and forces that are shaping modern civilization are better equipped to study themselves. To understand yourself, you must also understand the world you live in. You don't have to become an intellectual (unless you happen to be one), but studying of the various components of human nature is wonderful mental training, and it can help you thoroughly comprehend the wisdom of Yoga.

Relating to a higher principle

The third element of self-restraint *(niyama)* is devotion to a higher principle. The Sanskrit term is *ishvara-pranidhana,* where the word *ishvara* means "lord," referring to the divine. We translate it as "higher principle" to emphasize that you don't need to believe in a personal God to perform this practice. Devotion to a higher principle essentially means keeping your sight fixed on realizing your highest spiritual potential. If you happen to believe in a personal deity, you can use the traditional practice of repeating whatever name you have for the divine until your mind becomes absorbed in the state of contemplation. Or you can employ prayers and invocations to feel near to God or Goddess. But always remember that, according to Yoga, the divine isn't a separate being but the essence of everything.

Chapter 21

Meditation and the Higher Reaches of Yoga

You've probably heard the saying, "You give as good as you get." The same goes for Yoga. Doing a few postures now and then certainly gives you some benefits; however, to reap Yoga's full rewards, you need to live a yogic lifestyle — a lifestyle that encompasses the physical, mental, and spiritual.

Yoga postures are a great place to start. Combined with a decent diet, Yoga postures take care of 80 percent of your physical well-being and also have a positive effect on your emotional health. (The other 20 percent comes from adequate sleep, meaningful work, and a reasonably happy family life.)

Beyond the basic benefits of a healthy body, the physical practice of Yoga can help you continue to explore your deeper mental and spiritual potential. In fact, a vital, healthy body is the best foundation for meditation (yogic concentration) and the higher reaches of Yoga. Try meditating when your nose is blocked from a cold, when you're running a fever, or when your back is killing you. Pain and discomfort may make you philosophical ("Why me?"), but they don't contribute to a basically relaxed mind. And that's exactly why you need to meditate.

Many chapters in this book deal specifically with Yoga postures, which are designed to relax your body and thus prepare your mind for the higher stages of Yoga. This chapter explains how to integrate meditation into your routine so that you can reach the top rung of the Yoga ladder.

Understanding Concentration

How busy is your mind? Can you concentrate easily? The following little exercise gauges your CQ (Concentration Quotient):

Think of a beautiful white swan. It looks neither left nor right but just slowly and majestically glides across the surface of a pond. It barely causes ripples in the water. Just keep thinking of that swan. Try to form a clear image and then hold it as steadily as possible in your mind while slowly counting down from 100.

How far did you manage to count before your mental image of the swan faded into thin air or another thought intruded? Was it 97 or 96? Perhaps you lost your concentration with the count of 99. You may have been able to continue your counting for several more numbers, but reaching much beyond 96 is unusual for most beginners. If you did, your power of concentration is good — only a yogi or yogini can count all the way to 0 and think of the swan.

If you think you didn't do well with this exercise because visualizing isn't your strong suit, try this one for good measure:

Sit quietly. Take a few deep breaths and then let your mind go totally blank. No thoughts, no images, no counting — no ripples in your mental pond at all. Just sit. Just be.

How did you do? Don't feel bad if your concentration exercise went something like this:

". . . Okay, I'm not thinking. Heck, that's a thought, isn't it? Let me try again. . . . That's much better. See? Having no images isn't that difficult. And what was that about counting? I didn't do too well with the counting test, but I hate tests. Oh darn, I'm thinking again. Okay, back to no thoughts. . . ."

Don't be discouraged if your mind is a veritable speed train and your concentration is too poor to slow it down. Your mind's forward charge merely means that you have room for improvement, and you *will* improve with practice. Distraction isn't negative in itself. Instead, you can look at your lack of clear concentration as an opportunity to gently refocus your attention. As you refocus repeatedly, your mind can become more obedient. Think of your mind as a spirited foal that exuberantly gallops around the meadow. With a little training, that frisky colt can become an excellent racehorse. The following sections delve into how concentration works and what it can do for you.

Unleashing your essence

The ability to concentrate is a boon to everything you do. Without it, you'd constantly hammer your finger rather

The inner limbs of Yoga

According to Raja Yoga, as described in the *Yoga-Sutra* of Patanjali, the yogic path comprises eight limbs *(anga)*. The first five limbs — moral discipline, self-restraint, posture, breath control, and sensory inhibition — are called *outer limbs*. These practices belong to the entrance hall of Yoga's vast mansion. In the interior of the estate you find concentration, meditation, and ecstasy, known as the *inner limbs.* You can successfully practice these inner limbs only after you achieve a certain degree of mastery in the other five practices.

than a nail, you'd miscalculate your taxes, and you'd be unable to follow the razor-sharp logic of Sherlock Holmes.

Yogic concentration is far more demanding than the kind of concentration you use in daily life; but it's also much more rewarding. Yoga can help you unlock the hidden chambers of your own mind. When you're able to focus your attention on your inner world like a laser, you can discover the most subtle aspects of your mind. Above all, yogic concentration ultimately enables you to discover your spiritual essence.

Concentration leads to meditation (which we discuss later in the chapter) and brings you clarity and peace of mind — two qualities that stand you in good stead in any situation. They enable you to live your life more fully, more meaningfully, and more competently. Whether you're a busy mother and homemaker or a top executive, the mental tranquility you produce through regular concentration and meditation exercises can transform your entire day.

Gaining focus

Concentration and meditation are special moments in the same mindfulness that you're asked to bring to every aspect of your life. The Sanskrit word for *concentration* is *dharana,* which means "holding." You hold your attention by focusing on a specific bodily process (such as breathing), a thought, an image, or a sound (as we discuss in "Practicing Meditation" later in the chapter). Through *concentration,* you seek to become *concentric,* or properly centered and harmonious with yourself. When you're out of center *(eccentric),* or out of touch with your spiritual core, all your thoughts and actions are out of sync; they don't flow from your innermost core and thus make you feel alienated, uneasy, and unhappy.

You can determine whether you're currently *concentric* or *eccentric* by checking in with your body. How do you feel? How does a decision you're about to make feel? How does a relationship feel? What does your body tell you about your present activity or your job? How do you feel about your life as a whole? This kind of mindfulness is called *focusing,* which means paying careful attention to how your mind is registering in your body. Body and mind go together, so keeping mentally in touch with your body regularly is vital and even fundamental to good postural practice.

Through focusing, you can also become aware of your own baggage — old resentments, disappointments, fears, and expectations. People tend to store negative experiences in their bodies, which makes them predisposed to sickness. Sooner or later, each person needs to work through these stored memories for their own good health and to share their liberated selves with the world around them.

One way to begin replaying and diffusing negative experiences that are recorded in your body is to ask yourself, "Is anything preventing me from feeling good and happy right now? What, if anything, is keeping me from experiencing bliss?" Your body contains the answer(s): a sensation of tightness in the chest, a hollow feeling around the heart, a contraction in the pit of your stomach, fearful pounding in the head — you get the idea. All these reactions are physical expressions of corresponding emotional states.

 When doing this kind of focusing work, don't settle for the first answer that comes to mind. Instead, ask yourself, "What else is there to prevent me from feeling good and happy?" If you encounter too much inner pain, you may want to consider doing this work in the company of a trusted friend or under the guidance of a competent counselor or therapist.

Practicing Meditation

Meditation is a mental process involving focused attention (also known as *calm awareness* or *mindfulness*). Many people confuse meditation with stopping all thoughts, but that's only one (rather advanced) type of meditation. In the beginning, meditation is simply noticing the endless stream of thoughts flickering on your mental screen; consider your observations an important part of your overall effort to be *mindful,* or attentive.

Many forms or styles of meditation exist, but two basic approaches stand out: *meditation with a specific focus* and *objectless meditation*. The latter is pure mindfulness without narrowing attention to any particular sensation, idea, or other phenomenon. Most beginners find this kind of meditation very difficult, although some are drawn to it. We recommend that you start out with meditation on a specific focus. The following categories of objects are suitable for this exercise:

- ✔ A bodily sensation, such as breathing, which makes an excellent focus

- ✔ A bodily location, such as one of the seven cakras or energy centers we discuss in the next section

- ✔ A process or action, such as eating, walking, or washing dishes

- ✔ An external physical object, such as the flame of a candle

- ✔ A *mantra* (be it a single sound, a phrase, or a chant)

- ✔ A thought, such as the idea of peace, joy, love, or compassion

- ✔ A visualization of light, emptiness, a saint, or one of the many deities of Hindu or Buddhist Yoga

 Experiment with all these various focal points for meditation until you find what appeals to you the most. Then stick with it. For instance, if you choose to visualize a particular saint or deity, you benefit by always using the same figure in your daily visualization practice.

The following sections give you more information on mastering meditation.

Getting a handle on cakras: Your wheels of fortune

If you choose to focus your meditation on a cakra (one of the options in the earlier list), you first need to understand the concept of cakras. According to Yoga, the physical body has a more subtle energetic counterpart that consists of a network of energy channels called *nadis* (pronounced *nah-dees*) through which the life force *(prana)* circulates. The most important channel, called the *sushumna-nadi* or "gracious channel," runs along the axis of the body from the base of the spine to the crown of the head. In the ordinary individual, this central conduit of subtle energy is said to be mostly inactive. The purpose of many Hatha Yoga exercises is to clear this channel in particular of any obstructions, so that the life energy can flow freely in it, leading to better health and also higher states of consciousness.

When the central channel is thus activated, it also sets the seven psychoenergetic centers of the body in motion. These centers are the *cakras* (often spelled *chakras* in English), which are aligned along the central channel. The word means simply "wheel" and refers to the fact that these areas are whirlpools of energy that keep the physical body alive and functioning properly. In ascending order, the seven cakras are

- **Muladhara ("root prop," pronounced *moo-lahd-hah-rah*):** Located at the base of the spine between the rectum and genitals, this center is the resting place of the dormant "serpent power," the great psychospiritual energy that Hatha Yoga seeks to awaken. This center is connected with elimination as well as fear.

- **Svadhishthana ("own place," pronounced *svahd-hisht-hah-nah*):** Located at the genitals, this center is connected with the urogenital functions but also with desire.

- **Manipura ("jewel city," pronounced *mah-nee-poo-rah*):** Located at the navel, this center distributes the life force to all parts of the body and is especially involved in the digestive process as well as the willpower.

- *Anahata* (**"unstruck," pronounced** *ah-nah-hah-tah*): Located in the middle of the chest, this center, which is also called the "heart cakra," is the place where the "unstruck" or inner sound can be heard in meditation. It's also linked with love.

- *Vishuddha* (**"pure," pronounced** *vee-shood-hah*): Located at the throat, this center is associated with speech as well as greed.

- *Ajna* (**"command," pronounced** *ah-gyah*): Located in the middle of the head between the eyebrows, this center is the contact place for the *guru's* telepathic work with disciples. It's also associated with the experience of higher states of consciousness.

- *Sahasrara* (**"thousand-spoked," pronounced** *sah-hahs-rah-rah*): Located at the crown of the head, this special cakra is associated with higher states of consciousness, notably the ecstatic state (which we cover in "Working toward Ecstasy" later in the chapter).

Following a few guidelines for successful meditation

Think of your meditation as a tree that you must water every day — not too much and not too little. Trust that one day your nurturing will bring the tree to bear beautiful blossoms and delicious fruit.

Here are several vital tips to help you set the stage for a meditation routine:

- **Practice regularly.** Try to meditate every day. If that isn't possible, meditate at least several times a week.

- **Cultivate the correct motivation.** People meditate for all kinds of reasons: health, wholeness, peace of mind, clarity, spiritual growth, and so on. Be clear in your own mind why you're sitting down to meditate. The best motivation for meditation (and Yoga practice in general) is to live to your full potential *and* to benefit others by your personal achievements.

In Buddhism, this motivation is known as the *bodhisattva* ideal. The *bodhisattva* ("enlightenment being") seeks to realize enlightenment (the ultimate spiritual state) for the benefit of all other beings. As an enlightened being, you can be far more efficient in helping others in their own struggle for wholeness and happiness.

- **Meditate at a regular time.** Take advantage of the fact that your body-mind is a creature of habit. After a few weeks of meditating at the same time during the day or night, you may find yourself looking forward to your next meditation session. Traditionally, Yoga practitioners prefer the hour of sunrise, but this time isn't always practical. (Head to Chapter 18 for more on morning meditation.)

Inevitably, you have moments when meditation is the last thing you want to do. In that case, resolve to sit quietly for at least five minutes. Often, this break is enough to get you in the mood for full-fledged meditation. If not, don't beat yourself over the head; just go on to something else and try again later or the next day.

- ✔ **Meditate in the same place.** Choose the same place for the same reason you use the same time: Your body-mind enjoys what is familiar. Use this fact to your advantage by setting aside a room or a corner of a room that your mind can associate with meditation.

- ✔ **Select an appropriate posture for meditation and do it correctly.** Sit up straight, with your chest open, and your neck free (see the following section for instructions about posture). To avoid falling asleep, don't recline while meditating and don't meditate on your bed, even in a sitting position, because your mind is likely to associate the experience with sleep. If you're not used to sitting on the floor, try sitting on a straight-backed chair or on a sofa with a cushion behind your back. If you can comfortably sit on the floor, you have a variety of yogic postures to choose from, several of which appear in Chapter 7.

- ✔ **Select a meditation technique and stick with it.** In the beginning, you may want to try out various techniques to see which appeals to you the most. But after you find a good technique for your particular needs, don't abandon it until it bears fruit (in terms of increased peace of mind and happiness), a meditation teacher advises you to change to a different technique, or you feel really drawn to a different technique.

When you have your routine sorted out, keep the following suggestions in mind as you grow your meditation tree:

- ✔ **Begin with short sessions.** Meditate only 10 to 20 minutes at a time at first. If your meditation naturally lasts longer, simply rejoice in the fact. But never force yourself if the timing creates conflict or unhappiness in you. Also, beware of overmeditating. Often, what beginners regard as a nice long meditation is just self-indulgent daydreaming. Make sure that your meditation contains an element of alertness. When you start drifting off into a comfortable space, you can be sure that you're no longer meditating. Like the practice of the Yoga postures, your meditation must have an *edge* (that is, you must push against the limitations of your mind but without frustrating yourself).

✔ **Be alert, yet relaxed.** Inner alertness, or mindfulness, isn't the same as tension or stress. Cats are good examples of this alertness. Even when a cat is completely relaxed, its ears move around like radar dishes catching every little sound in the environment. The more relaxed you are, the more alert your mind can be, so make sure that your body is relaxed by regularly practicing some of the relaxation exercises we describe in Chapter 4.

✔ **Don't burden yourself with expectations.** Entering meditation with a desire to grow spiritually and to benefit from the experience is certainly acceptable. However, don't expect every meditation to be wonderful and pleasant.

✔ **Prepare properly for meditation.** As a beginner, don't expect to be able to jump from the fray of your daily activities straight into meditation. Allow your mind a little time to unwind before you sit for meditation. Have a relaxing bath or shower or at least wash your face and hands.

✔ **At the end of your meditation, integrate the experience with the rest of your life.** Just as going straight from overdrive into a meditative gear isn't prudent, you need to refrain from jumping up from meditation to return to your other activities. Instead, make a conscious transition in and out of meditation. At the end of the session, briefly recall your reasons for meditating and your overall motivation. Be grateful for any energies and/or insights your meditation generates. Equally importantly, don't feel negative about a difficult meditation experience. Rather, be grateful for *any* experience. Sometimes important insights surface during meditation, and then your challenge is to translate these messages into daily life. When you continually perform this kind of integration, your meditation deepens more quickly as well.

✔ **Be prepared to practice meditation for a lifetime.** You don't grow a tree overnight. On the yogic path, no effort is ever wasted. Therefore, don't give up if your meditation isn't what you think it should be after a month or two. Don't conclude too hastily that meditation isn't working or that the technique you're using isn't effective. Instead, correct your understanding about the nature of meditation and carry on. Your very effort to meditate counts.

Be wary of weekend workshops that promise immediate success, if not enlightenment itself. Meditation and enlightenment are lifelong processes.

Maintaining proper bodily posture

Correct posture is important for meditation. Here's a seven-point checklist that can help you develop good sitting habits:

Roses come with thorns

If you're a beginner and your meditations are consistently comfortable, you have every reason to be suspicious. The purpose of meditation is to clear your mind, and doing so entails clearing away the debris (or what one teacher has called "the frogs deep down in the well").

In the beginning, meditation consists largely of discovering just how unruly your mind is. If your meditation practice is successful, you encounter your shadow side (all those aspects of your character you'd prefer not to think about). As you go on, more profound insights into your character can and do occur, which then requires you to make the necessary changes in your attitudes and behaviors.

Few meditations are spectacular, which isn't at all what meditation is about. Even a seemingly bad meditation is a good meditation because you're applying mindfulness. Don't be surprised to find that your meditation is calm and uplifting one day and turbulent and distracted the next for no apparent reason. Until your mind reaches clarity and calmness, you can expect this fluctuation. Just keep a sense of humor and graciously accept whatever happens in your meditation.

✔ **Back:** Your back position is the single most important physical feature of your meditation. Your back should be straight but relaxed, with your chest open and your neck free. Correct posture enables your bodily energies to flow more freely, which prevents sleepiness. (Flip to "Understanding cakras: Your wheels of fortune" earlier in the chapter for details on the bodily energies.) Most Westerners need a firm cushion under their *sits bones* (the bones directly under the flesh of the buttocks) to encourage good posture during meditation and to stop their legs from going to sleep. If you go that route, however, make sure your pelvis doesn't tilt forward too much. Alternatively, you can sit on a chair. Any posture is acceptable as long as you can comfortably maintain it for the desired duration.

✔ **Head:** For the correct position of your head, picture an attached string pulling the back of your head upward so that your head is tilted slightly forward. Too much of a forward tilt invites drowsiness, but not enough of a tilt can cause mental wandering.

✔ **Tongue:** Allow the front part of your tongue to touch the palate just behind the upper teeth. This position reduces the flow of saliva and the number of times you have to swallow, which many beginners find disturbing.

✔ **Teeth:** Don't clench your teeth — keep your jaws relaxed. And be sure that your mouth doesn't hang open either.

✔ **Legs:** If you can sit cross-legged for an extended period of time without experiencing discomfort, we especially recommend the perfect posture (*siddhasana*), which we describe in Chapter 6. The folded legs form a closed circuit, which aids your concentration. If sitting cross-legged is a problem for you, just meditate in a chair.

✔ **Arms:** Keep your hands cupped in your lap with your palms up and your right hand on top of your left. Relax your arms and shoulders, leaving a few inches between your arms and your trunk, which allows the air to circulate and prevents drowsiness.

- **Eyes:** Most beginners like to close their eyes, which is fine. As you develop your power of concentration, however, you may want to experiment with keeping your eyes slightly open while gazing downward in front of you to signal your brain that you aren't trying to go to sleep. Advanced practitioners are able to keep their eyes wide open without becoming distracted. In any event, make sure that your eye muscles are relaxed.

Overcoming obstacles to meditation

Whenever you deal with change, you also deal with resistance to change. Thus, the path of meditation is littered with various obstacles that can trip you up. Here are the most important potential hindrances: doubt (about the yogic path or yourself), negative thoughts (about yourself, others, life, and so on), haste, boredom, pretense, and hunting for spiritual experiences. The ego lurks in many niches, especially when you travel on the yogic path.

Adding sounds to meditation

Using a sound or phrase to focus the mind is a popular approach in many spiritual traditions, including Hinduism, Buddhism, Christianity, Judaism, and Islamic Sufism. In Sanskrit, these special sounds are called *mantras* and are thought to help better focus attention. Mantra Yoga made its debut in the Western world in the late 1960s with the Transcendental Meditation (TM) movement, founded by Maharishi Mahesh Yogi, whose most famous disciples were The Beatles.

Here are some well-known *mantras:*

- The syllable *om* is composed of the letters *a, u,* and *m,* and stands for the waking state, dream state, and deep sleep respectively. Hindus consider this syllable to be sacred and to symbolize the ultimate reality, or higher Self *(atman).* The sound begins from the belly and moves upward; the long-drawn, nasalized humming sound of *m* represents the ultimate reality.

- The mantra *so'ham* (pronounced *so-hum*) means "I am He," that is, "I am the universal Self." You repeat it in sync with breathing: *so* on inhaling and *ham* on exhaling.

- Buddhist Yoga widely uses the mantric phrase *om mani padme hum* (pronounced *om mah-nee pahd-meh hoom*). It means *"Om.* Jewel in the Lotus. *Hum,"* which conveys that the searched-for higher reality is present here and now.

- The mantric utterance *om namah shivaya* (pronounced *om nah-mah shee-vah-yah*) is a favorite phrase among Hindu devotees of the Divine in the form of Shiva. It means *"Om.* Salutation to Shiva."

- The mantric utterance *hare krishna* (pronounced *hah-reh krish-nah*) was made famous in the West by the members of the Krishna Consciousness movement. It invokes the Divine in the form of Krishna, who is also called Hari.

According to the Yoga tradition, sounds are considered mantras only after a guru passes the sound to a worthy disciple. Thus, the syllable *om* on its own — without proper initiation — isn't a mantra. Many Western Yoga teachers take a more relaxed approach and recommend both traditional and contemporary words for mantra practice.

Reciting your mantra

Whether you choose your own *mantra* or are given one, you must repeat it over and over again, either mentally or vocally (whispered or aloud), in order to make it effective.

This practice of recitation is called *japa* (pronounced *jah-pah*), meaning "muttering." So, what happens after you recite a *mantra* a thousand, ten thousand, or a hundred thousand times? As you repeat the sound, your attention becomes more and more focused and your consciousness becomes absorbed into the sound. The *mantra* begins to recite itself, serving as an anchor for your mind whenever you don't need to engage your thoughts in specific tasks. This shift simplifies your inner life and gives you a sense of peace. Ultimately, your *mantra* can guide you to enlightenment. Of course, to achieve enlightenment you must fulfill the other requirements of Yoga as well, notably honoring the moral disciplines, which we cover in detail in Chapter 18. We also discuss the road to enlightenment further in "Reaching toward Enlightenment" later in this chapter.

We recommend that beginners recite their mantra aloud, at a slow, steady pace. After you have some experience with this form of meditation, you can begin to whisper your mantra so that only you can hear it. Traditionally, the most powerful form of mantric recitation is silent or mental recitation. This exercise, however, calls for a certain degree of skill in maintaining your concentration, so start with a vocal mantra.

Using a rosary

Yoga practitioners often tell rosary beads while reciting their mantras — a practice that helps focus the mind. The typical rosary *(mala)* consists of 108 beads plus an extra-large bead that represents the cosmic mountain Meru.

You tell the beads by using the thumb and middle finger. Your fingers should not cross the master or Meru bead. After 108 recitations (or beads), you simply turn the rosary around and start counting over again.

Breathing mindfully

Mindful observation of the breath is a meditation exercise, taught particularly in Buddhist circles, that any beginner can try. As we note in Chapter 5, the breath is the link between body and mind and since ancient times, the Yoga masters have made good use of this connection. Mindful breathing, or breathing meditation, is a simple and effective way of exploring the calming effect of conscious breathing. Here's how it works:

1. **Sit up straight and relaxed.**

2. **Remind yourself of your purpose for meditation and resolve to sit in meditation for a given period of time.**

   We recommend at least 5 minutes for this exercise. Gradually extend the duration.

3. **Close your eyes or keep them half open while looking down in front of you.**

4. **Breathing normally and gently, focus your attention on the sensation created by the breath flowing in and out of your nostrils.**

   Carefully observe the entire process of inhalation and exhalation as it occurs at the opening of your nostrils.

5. **To prevent your mind from wandering, you can count in inhalation/exhalation breath cycles**

from 1 to 10.

Note: Don't be concerned if you notice that your attention has wandered. Especially, don't be judgmental about any thoughts that may pop into your head. Instead, rededicate yourself to the process of observing your breath.

Walking meditation

Mindfulness is possible in any circumstance. You can eat, drive, wash dishes, have a conversation, watch television, or make love mindfully. For beginners, mindfulness while walking is an excellent form of meditation. Just follow these steps to get started:

1. **Remind yourself of your purpose for meditation and resolve to meditate for a given period of time.**

    For a first try, we recommend at least 5 minutes for this exercise.

2. **Keep your eyes open but unfocused, looking down and a few steps ahead of you.**

    Don't lower your head, but keep your neck relaxed.

Associating prayer with meditation

A close relationship exists between meditation and prayer. Prayer practices mindfulness in relationship to a being — whether that be a *guru,* a great master (dead or alive), a deity, or the ultimate spiritual reality itself — deemed "higher" than the participant. Prayer, like meditation, involves a feeling of reverence.

3. **Stand completely still and feel your entire body.**

4. **Focus your attention on your right foot, especially the toes and sole.**

5. **Slowly raise your right foot and take the first step.**

   Feel the sensation of the pressure lifting from your right foot and leg and shifting over to your left leg.

6. **As you slowly place the right foot back on the ground, become aware of the contact between your sole and the ground.**

   Also notice the rest of your body: your swinging arms that keep you balanced, your neck and head, your pelvis.

7. **Acknowledge any thoughts that arise without being judgmental; return your attention to your whole body, not merely on one limb or movement.**

8. **At the end of your walking meditation, stand completely still for a few seconds, observing the clarity and calmness within you.**

Working toward Ecstasy

When you start meditating, you're well aware that "you" — the subject — are quite different from the object of meditation. You experience the white or blue light or the visualized deity as distinct from yourself. But as meditation deepens, the boundary between subject and object — consciousness and its contents — becomes increasingly blurred. Then, at one point, the two merge completely. You're the light

Wherever you go, there you are

Sri Ramana Maharshi was one of the great Yoga masters of the 20th century. When, as he was on his deathbed, his disciples expressed their sorrow at losing him, he calmly said, "They say that I am dying, but I am not going away. Where could I go? I am here." He had realized the eternal Self, which is everywhere. To this day, his spiritual presence can be felt in the hermitage that disciples built for him long ago.

or deity. This point is the celebrated state of ecstasy called *samadhi* in Sanskrit (pronounced *sah-mahd-hee*).

Yoga distinguishes two fundamental types or levels of ecstasy. At the lower level, the ecstatic state is associated with a certain form or mental content. The higher type of ecstasy is a state of formless consciousness.

Many Yoga practitioners never experience the ecstatic state, but some definitely encounter it in the course of their lives. What matters isn't how often or how long you enter into *samadhi* but whether and how much you embody spiritual principles in your daily life. Are you compassionate and kind? Do you see others not as total strangers but fellow beings going through their own struggle of Self-realization? Can you love unconditionally? Are you forgiving and encouraging toward others?

Samadhi isn't identical with enlightenment, which is the real goal of Yoga. You can attain enlightenment without ever experiencing *samadhi*. The following section enlightens you about the state of enlightenment.

480

Reaching toward Enlightenment

People usually associate the word *enlightenment* with profound intellectual understanding. However, in Yoga, enlightenment refers to the permanent realization of your true nature, which is the ultimate or transcendental Self *(atman)*. The Sanskrit word for enlightenment is *bodha* (pronounced *bohd-ha*), which means "illumination." The same realization also is referred to as *liberation* because it liberates you from the misunderstanding that you're a separate self, referred to as *I* in a unique body and gifted with a mind that is disconnected from everything else.

Chapter 22

Yoga Therapy: The (Yoga) Doctor Will See You Now

- -

In This Chapter

▶ Understanding Yoga therapy

▶ Following a five-step plan to keep your back shipshape

▶ Trying Yoga routines for lower backs and upper backs/necks

- -

Yoga therapy applies the principles of Yoga to people with physical, psychological, or spiritual needs not normally met in a group class. A *Yoga therapist* is a Yoga teacher with advanced training who can adapt Yoga to the client's unique needs. The regular and mindful practice of carefully adapted Yoga postures can bring relief from pain, increase mobility and strength, and confer a sense of well-being.

This chapter introduces you to the field of Yoga therapy, helps you make informed decisions about whether Yoga therapy may be right for you, and shows you what to look for in a Yoga therapist. If your back is calling for more TLC (but not crying out for a doctor — if you're in acute pain, see your medical professional), the suggestions and postures in this chapter can help you become more aware of your needs and make peace with your back.

What You Need to Know about Yoga Therapy

If you have ever suffered from a back problem, you aren't alone. More than 80 percent of Americans seek professional help for back pain at some point in their lives, and back pain is second only to the common cold for illness-related absences from work. Back-health experts recommend that people learn how to prevent pain and self-treat in situations where they can safely do so.

Yoga therapy helps people in the chronic or rehabilitation stage of their pain (after the acute stage has passed) and is generally an adjunct to medical and/or chiropractic care. Acute pain is the body's distress signal and shouldn't be ignored. What may feel like a musculoskeletal pain may in fact be a serious medical problem involving an organ, or a pinched nerve requiring spinal adjustment. People with acute pain should seek help from a medical, chiropractic, or osteopathic physician or physical therapist.

In addition to its most common use with back problems, Yoga therapy is helpful with knee and hip problems, arthritis, and carpal tunnel syndrome. It can also benefit those who suffer from a host of other conditions: heart disease, hypertension, insomnia, painful menstrual periods and hot flashes, depression, anxiety, headaches, diabetes, digestive problems, chronic pain, Parkinson's disease, multiple sclerosis, and more. Though not a cure, Yoga therapy can help improve the quality of life for people living with serious chronic and progressive conditions.

Everything old is new again: The evolution of Yoga as therapy

The therapeutic use of Yoga dates back over thousands of years as a component of *ayurveda*. *Ayurveda* (*ayus* meaning "life" and *veda* meaning "related to knowledge or science") is an Indian system of medicine with ancient roots that is becoming well known in the West as well. It has a strong focus on disease prevention and takes a whole-person approach. Yoga therapy came into its own in India in the early part of the 20th century. Sri T. Krishnamacacharya, teacher to T.K.V. Desikachar, B.K.S. Iyengar, and Pattabhi Jois, used his own blend of Yoga and *ayurveda*. The Kaivalyadhama Yoga Hospitalin Lonovola (www.kdham.com) and the Yoga Institute of Santacruz, Mumbai (www.theyogainstitute. org), both started almost a century ago and still operate today.

Yoga therapy has continued to develop in the United States, sometimes combined with ayurveda but increasingly utilized as a complement to Western-style integrative medicine. Early pioneers in the field include Dean Ornish, MD; Nischala Devi; Judith Lasater, PT; Gary Kraftsow, MA; your humble coauthors Georg Feuerstein, PhD and Larry Payne, PhD; Michael Lee; Richard Miller, PhD; and Makunda Stiles. Founded in 1989 by Richard Miller and me (Larry), the International Association of Yoga Therapists (www.iayt.org) supports research and education in Yoga and serves as a professional organization for upward of 2,600 Yoga therapists and teachers worldwide.

If you think you may be a candidate for Yoga therapy, the next step is to find a qualified Yoga therapist who can meet your needs. The following sections help you with that search and also clue you in as to what you can expect from Yoga therapy.

How to find a good Yoga therapist

Finding a good Yoga therapist who fits your needs takes a bit of research. Following are some tips that should help you in you in your search:

- ✔ **Find out where the Yoga therapist has received training.** Look for someone who has successfully completed a respected training program. The Yoga Therapy Rx training program at Loyola Marymount University in Los Angeles is the first of what is sure to become many university-based programs to prepare Yoga teachers to apply the tools of Yoga to bring relief and improvement. We also list other highly respected non-university programs, some with specific specialties in the appendix.

- ✔ **Ask a trusted source.** Yoga therapists work with a range of health care practitioners. Ask your practitioner for a referral.

- ✔ **Visit the Web site of a respected training program.** Many training programs publish the names and contact information of therapists they have trained. While at the site, you can explore the training course descriptions and evaluate their appropriateness for your needs.

What to expect if you see a Yoga therapist

Visiting any new practitioner can make a person uneasy, so in this section, we guide you to be an informed patient, discussing the Yoga therapy approach to healing as well as treatment length and cost.

A whole-person approach

Yoga therapy takes the whole person into account. Although your chief complaint may be your achin' lower back, in the course of the assessment your Yoga therapist may observe, ask about, and consider related factors beyond your tense muscles: how and how much you move and sit during the course of your typical day; your general level of stress (without becoming your psychotherapist); how you breathe; your typical diet and sleep patterns; and so on. In addition to an individualized program of coordinated movement and breath, your Yoga therapist may suggest journaling to help you learn more about your lifestyle and pain triggers as well as modifications in your daily routine to help you meet your goal.

An initial series of sessions, and beyond

About six sessions are generally helpful when working with a Yoga therapist. This duration allows time for you to get a handle on your personalized program, and for your Yoga therapist to observe and adjust your movements and breath so that you have a program that works for you.

The goal is to develop a personal practice that you can continue on your own for continued improvement in mobility, strength, and well-being so that you can eventually participate in group classes if you want to. Periodic tune-ups are a good idea, especially if you aren't participating in a group class where a skilled Yoga teacher can help you modify postures as necessary.

Cost

As you may expect, private sessions with someone who has advanced training cost more than what you'd pay for a group Yoga class. Individual sessions in large metropolitan areas range from about \$75 to \$200 each depending on the experience of the therapist.

Five-Step Plan for a Healthy Back

The best way to prevent back problems or to keep them from becoming chronic is to use Yoga as part of a five-step plan, which we outline here.

- ✔ **Re-educate yourself on biomechanics:** How you sit, stand, walk, lift, sleep, and work can cause you pain or help you relieve pain.

- ✔ **Practice your Yoga or back exercise program regularly:** Be realistic about how much you can do each day, and *do it.*

- ✔ **Keep a back journal:** Journaling can help you discover more about how your lifestyle (such as sleeping, lifting, and sitting habits) affects your back.

- ✔ **Make healthful food choices:** Nutrition experts recommend a balanced diet rich in fruits and vegetables, whole grains, legumes, low fat dairy products, fish, and limited amounts of lean meat, if meat is eaten.

- ✔ **Rest and relax consciously:** Be mindful about what you expose yourself to in the hours before bedtime. The last thing you see or listen to before bed affects your subconscious mind and can affect your sleep pattern.

Yoga Rx for Lower Backs

Your "lower back" is actually the *lumbar vertebrae* section of the spinal cord. Spine movement brings much-needed circulation to the vertebral discs and helps keep them supple. The health of your hamstring and *psoas* (hip flexor) muscles as well as the strength of your abdominal and core muscles also affects your lower back. Helpful Yoga therapy postures allow you to stretch and strengthen key muscle groups, release tension and bring your whole body back into harmony. The following sections give you some general guidelines on what kinds of Yoga movements work well for different lower back issues, and a routine to help you segue into a regular group class.

Lower back conditions that need more arching

If a forward bend or rounding is very painful to your lower back, chances are you may have strained your lower back muscles or may have a disc problem or sciatica. So, be wise, and if it hurts, don't do it! Here are some tips:

- ✔ **Avoid forward bends of any kind.** If you try a forward bend, keep your back flat and not rounded. Remember the concept of Forgiving Limbs (which we cover in Chapter 3) and bend your knees as necessary.

- ✔ **Try postures that allow you to arch, such as those in the cobra family (see Chapter 11), rather than bend forward.** Gentle extensions such as transitioning to warrior I from the mountain posture are also helpful. (Check out Chapter 7 for warrior I and mountain posture.)

- ✔ **Use the "Lower back routine" later in this section.** You can also find DVD resources in the appendix.

Lower back conditions that need more folding

A number of back conditions, including arthritis and *spondylolisthesis* (slipped vertebrae), can cause the vertebrae to jam, making arching very painful. As we stress in the preceding section, if it hurts, don't do it. The following list gives you some pointers on Yoga for these conditions:

✔ Avoid postures that extend your back, such as those in the cobra family, and athletic postures or sequences that involve jumping.

✔ Try postures that lengthen your back, such as gentle forward bends, downward-facing dog, and folding cat. (Flip to Chapter 7 for more suggestions.)

What about scoliosis?

Scoliosis, a condition where the spine curves from side to side, can be structural or functional. If you feel you have scoliosis, consult with your medical or chiropractic physician.

✔ *Structural scoliosis* is a hereditary disorder more common in girls than boys.

✔ *Functional scoliosis* may occur as a result of a problem elsewhere in the body, such as one leg being shorter than the other, or even as a result of very frequent holding of a position that causes a twist in the spine. Postures that stretch out one side of the spine at a time, such as *asymmetrical* (one-sided) forward bends, side bends, and twists are generally helpful and may reduce or eliminate the curve in time. (Chapters 11 and 12 give you more info on postures that bend and twist.)

Lower back routine

The following exercises aren't meant for acute back problems. If any part of this routine causes you back or neck pain, omit that part and check with your medical or chiropractic physician before you continue.

A session or two of Yoga or back exercise during your week doesn't help much if you misuse or abuse your back the rest of the time.

No single Yoga routine is appropriate for all back problems. When your doctor feels that you're ready for a regular group class, the following routine can help you make the transition. Keep in mind that the Yoga breathing we recommend for this routine (Chapter 5's focus breathing or belly breathing) is just as important as the Yoga postures. Inhale and exhale slowly through your nose, with a slight pause after both the inhalation and the exhalation. We give you various options for many of the postures so that you can find the moves that are right for you. And remember that executing the postures in the proper sequence is very important.

Corpse posture with bent legs: Shavasana variation

Relaxation and breathing are important ingredients for a healthy back. The corpse posture is a classic position to start the process.

If your back feels uncomfortable, place a pillow or blanket roll under your knees. If your head tilts back, place a folded blanket or small pillow under your head.

1. **Lie flat on your back with your arms relaxed along the sides of your torso and your palms up.**

2. Bend your knees and place your feet on the floor at hip width.

3. Close your eyes and relax (see Figure 22-1).

4. Stay in the posture for 8 to 10 breaths.

Figure 22-1: *Corpse posture with bent legs.*

Knee-to-chest posture: Ekapada apanasana

Keeping your back healthy is like tuning a piano. The knee-to-chest posture helps you adjust and relax your lower back. If you have knee problems, hold the back of your thigh instead of just below your knee. Remember, this pose isn't a biceps exercise. Just hold your knee, breathe, and relax.

1. Lie on your back with your knees bent palms down and feet flat on the floor.

2. As you exhale, bring your right knee toward your chest, holding your shin just below your knee as in Figure 22-2.

3. Stay in the posture for six to eight breaths.

4. Repeat Steps 1 through 3 with your left leg.

Figure 22-2:
Knee-to-chest posture.

Lying arm raise with bent leg: Shavasana variation

Many back sufferers have more problems on one side of the torso than the other. The lying arm raise is a safe, classic way to gently stretch and prepare each side of the back and neck for the rest of the routine.

1. **Lie in the corpse posture (found in Chapter 14) with your arms relaxed at your sides and palms down; bend just your left knee, and put your left foot on the floor as shown in Figure 22-3a.**

2. **As you inhale, slowly raise your arms overhead and touch the floor behind you with your palms up as Figure 22-3b illustrates; pause briefly.**

3. **As you exhale, bring your arms back to your sides as in Step 1.**

4. **Repeat Steps 2 and 3 six to eight times and then repeat Steps 1 through 3 with your right knee bent and your left leg straight.**

Figure 22-3:
Lying arm raise with bent leg.

Push-downs I: Urdhva prasrta padasana I

Note: We recommend that you start with this posture and replace it with push-downs II (in the following section) when you're ready to advance.

The abdomen is considered the front of your back (see Chapter 9). Keep this key area strong and toned if you want to prevent back problems. The push-downs are a great way to get that party started because they strengthen your abs without involving your neck and improve your core strength.

1. **Lying on your back with your knees bent and your feet on the floor at hip width, rest your arms near your sides with your palms down.**

2. **As you exhale, push your lower back down to the floor for 3 to 5 seconds as demonstrated in Figure 22-4 and then inhale.**

    As you inhale, your back releases from the push-down.

3. **Repeat Step 2 six to eight times.**

Figure 22-4: Push-downs I.

Push-downs II: Urdhva prasrta padasana II

When you're ready for push-downs II (the advanced version of push-downs I in the preceding section), move your bent leg very slowly. Resist the temptation to speed up.

1. **Lying on your back with your knees bent and your feet on the floor at hip width, rest your arms near your sides with your palms down.**

2. **As you inhale, draw your right bent knee in toward your chest, keeping your palms on the floor as in Figure 22-5.**

3. **As you exhale, push your lower back down to the floor, moving your bent right leg down until your right foot returns to touch the floor.**

   Repeat Steps 2 and 3 six to eight times, alternating slowly with right and left legs.

Figure 22-5:
Push-downs II.

To make push-downs II more challenging, draw both bent knees in toward your chest on the inhalation and then push your lower back into the floor as you bring both of your feet back to the floor on the exhalation. Be sure to keep both hands palms down on the floor the whole time.

Dynamic bridge: Dvipada pitham

The gentle action of the bridge compensates the abs and relaxes the back for the hamstring stretch in the following section. (Head to Chapter 15 for more on sequencing and compensation.)

1. **Lie on your back with your knees bent and feet flat on the floor at hip width.**

2. **Place your arms at your sides with your palms down.**

3. **As you inhale, raise your hips to a comfortable height as demonstrated in Figure 22-6.**

4. **As you exhale, return your hips to the floor.**

   Repeat Steps 3 and 4 six to eight times.

TIP

Try just tilting your pelvis towards your chin as you exhale if the bridge causes any problems, and then try the bridge again later when you're ready.

Figure 22-6: Dynamic bridge.

Hamstring stretch: Supta padangustasana variation

Tight hamstring muscles are a key factor in many cases of chronic back problems. A fine balance exists between stretching your hamstrings and not aggravating a chronic back condition. For this reason, we recommend keeping one leg bent with the foot on the floor to support your back.

1. **Lying on your back with your legs straight, place your arms along your sides with your palms down.**

2. **Bend just your left knee and put your left foot on the floor as in Figure 22-7a.**

3. **As you exhale, raise your right leg until it's perpendicular to the floor (or as close as you can manage).**

4. **As you inhale, return your leg to the floor, keeping your head and the top of your hips on the floor.**

   Repeat Steps 1 through 4 three to four times, and then hold the back of your raised thigh in place just below your knee for 6 to 8 breaths as in Figure 22-7b.

5. **Repeat Steps 1 through 4 on the other side with your right knee bent and your left leg straight.**

Make sure you feel the stretch in your hamstrings, not in your back.

If the back of your neck or your throat tenses when you raise or lower your leg, rest your head on a pillow or folded blanket.

Figure 22-7: Hamstring stretch.

Balancing cat: Chakravakasana variation I

This posture has been proven to strengthen core muscles throughout the spine, making it a great back exercise.

1. **Starting on your hands and knees, position your knees about hip width and your hands just below your shoulders with your fingers turned forward and your arms straightened as Figure 22-8a illustrates.**

2. **As you exhale, slide your right hand forward and your left leg back, keeping your hand and your toes on the floor.**

3. **As you inhale, raise your right arm and left leg to a comfortable height as in Figure 22-8b.**

4. **Stay in Step 3 for 6 to 8 breaths and then repeat Steps 1 through 3 with opposite pairs (left arm and right leg).**

Figure 22-8: Balancing cat posture.

497

To make this posture easier, keep both hands on the ground as you extend each leg.

Child's posture with arms in front: Balasana variation I

If you listen for feedback from your body after doing a number of back bends, you hear a clear desire to fold as compensation (which we cover in Chapter 15). The child's posture is a smooth and easy way to fold when you're concluding hands and knees postures or front-lying back bends. The arms-in-front variation here distributes the stretch along the upper and lower back.

1. **Starting on your hands and knees, place your knees about hip width with your hands just below your shoulders and your elbows straight but not locked.**

2. **As you exhale, sit back on your heels, rest your torso on your thighs, and place your forehead on the floor.**

3. **Lay your arms on the floor outstretched comfortably in front of you with your palms down as Figure 22-9 indicates.**

Close your eyes and breathe easily. Stay for 6 to 8 breaths.

Figure 22-9:
Child's posture
variation.

498

You can also try the regular child's posture with your arms back near your hips with your palms up and hands on the floor. You may feel a little more stretch in your lower back, so choose the one that's most comfortable in the moment.

 If you have knee or hip problems, lie on your back and do the knees-to-chest posture we cover later in this routine rather than the child's posture.

Half warrior: Ardha virabhadrasana variation

This posture stretches your main hip flexors (the *iliopsoas*), one of the key muscle groups for maintaining a healthy lower back.

1. **Start standing on your knees at hip width and then take a big step forward with the right foot, keeping your left knee on the ground; square your hips forward and place your hands on your right thigh, fingers forward just above your knee as shown in Figure 22-10a.**

2. **As you exhale, sink your hips forward and down as Figure 22-10b demonstrates.**

   Be sure to keep approximately a 90-degree angle with your forward leg.

3. **As you inhale return to the starting position in Step 1.**

4. **Repeat Steps 2 and 3 three to four times and then stay in Step 2 for six to eight breaths.**

5. **Repeat Steps 1 through 4 the same sequence on the left side.**

Figure 22-10: *Half warrior variation.*

Cobra II: Bhujangasana

Note: We recommend that you use either this posture or the cobra I posture in the following section, not both. Cobra I is less strenuous than cobra II, so go with cobra I if you aren't sure. Flip to Chapter 11 for further clarification.

As we explain in Chapter 11, most folks simply do too much forward bending. Finding a way to compensate with some form of back bend is important.

1. **Lie on your abdomen, with your legs at hip width and the tops of your feet on the floor.**

   You can also separate your legs further and roll your heels outward and toes inward.

2. **Bend your elbows and place your palms on the floor with your thumbs near your armpits.**

   Rest your forehead on the floor and relax your shoulders (see Figure 22-11a).

3. **As you inhale, press your palms against the floor and lift your chest and head forward and up (like a turtle coming out of its shell), keeping your buttocks loose.**

4. **Look straight ahead as shown in Figure 22-11b.**

   Keep the top front of your pelvis on the floor and your shoulders relaxed. Unless you're very flexible, keep your elbows slightly bent and roll them inward toward your trunk.

5. **As you exhale, lower your torso and head slowly back to the floor.**

   Repeat Steps 3 through 5 six to eight times.

Figure 22-11:
Cobra II.

Move slowly and cautiously in all of the cobra-like postures. Avoid any of the postures that cause pain in your lower back, upper back, or neck. If cobra II is too strenuous, use cobra I, which appears in the following section, or repeat the lying arm raise, which we cover earlier in this chapter.

Cobra I: Sphinx

Note: We recommend that you use either this posture or the cobra posture in the preceding section, not both. Cobra I is less strenuous than cobra II, so go with cobra I if you aren't sure.

If the cobra postures aggravate your lower back, separate your legs wider than your hips and turn your heels out with your toes inward. Also, if you move your hands further forward, these postures are less difficult.

1. **Lie on your abdomen with your legs at hip width and the tops of the feet on the floor.**

2. **Rest your forehead on the floor and relax your shoulders.**

   Bend your elbows and place your forearms on the floor with your palms turned down and positioned near the sides of your head.

3. **As you inhale, engage your back muscles, press your forearms against the floor, and raise your chest and head as in Figure 22-12.**

   Look straight ahead and keep your forearms and the front of your pelvis on the floor. Continue to relax your shoulders.

4. **As you exhale, lower your torso and head slowly back to the floor.**

5. **Repeat Steps 2 through 4 six to eight times.**

Figure 22-12:
Cobra I.

Prone resting posture Advasana variation

Resting at the right times is an important part of a Yoga sequence, and back bends may be the most strenuous part of your back routine. Remember, Yoga should never feel like you're in a hurry.

1. **Lie on your abdomen with your legs at hip**

width and the tops of your feet on the floor.

2. **Rest your forehead on the floor or turn your head to one side and relax your shoulders.**

Bend your elbows and place your forearms on the floor with your palms turned down and positioned near the sides of your head as shown in Figure 22-13. Stay for 6 to 8 breaths.

Figure 22-13:
Prone resting posture.

 If this resting position is uncomfortable for you, use the bent knee corpse posture we describe earlier in the chapter.

Locust I: Shalabhasana

The cobra postures in the preceding sections work primarily to stretch your back and restore its natural curves, but the locust posture works more on strengthening your back. Both are important to your back health.

1. **Lie on your abdomen with your legs at hip width and the tops of your feet on the floor.**

Rest your forehead on the floor.

2. **Extend your arms back along the sides of your torso with your palms on the floor.**

3. **As you inhale, raise your chest, head, and right leg as illustrated in Figure 22-14.**

503

4. **As you exhale, lower your torso and head slowly to the floor.**

5. **Repeat Steps 3 and 4 three times and then stay in Step 3 (the last raised position) for 6 to 8 breaths.**

6. **Repeat Steps 1 through 5 with your left leg.**

Figure 22-14:
The locust posture helps to strengthen your back and neck.

 If this posture is too strenuous for you, try it without lifting your leg or by just bending one leg at the knee with both thighs still on the ground.

Child's posture with arms back: Balasana variation II

Repeat the child's posture from earlier in the chapter, except keep your arms at your sides pointing back to your feet (see Figure 22-15).

Close your eyes and breathe easily. Stay for 6 to 8 breaths.

Figure 22-15:
Child's posture.

The butterfly: Jathara parvritti variation I

Back pain sufferers often forget that the lower and upper back are very connected. Often, an upper back twist like the butterfly has a safe ripple effect all the way down when a lower back twist isn't possible.

If you're having a disc-related problem, be very careful of twists for both the upper and lower back. If you have any negative symptoms, such as pain or numbness, leave the twist out and speak to your physician before adding it back into your program.

1. **Lie on your left side with your knees bent, arms extended parallel not higher than your shoulders and join your palms together on the floor as Figure 22-16a illustrates.**

   Place pillows or folded blankets under your head and between your knees for stability.

2. **As you inhale, raise your right hand up and over, turning your head to follow your hand until it touches the floor on the other side as in Figure 22-16b.**

   Don't force it! Only move your hand and head as far

as it can comfortably go.

3. **As you exhale, return to the starting position in Step 1.**

4. **Repeat Steps 2 and 3 four to six times.**

5. **Repeat Steps 1 through 4 on the right side.**

Figure 22-16:
The butterfly.

Bent-leg supine twist variation: Jathara parvritti variation II

A good back routine often includes both an upper and a lower back twist. The bent-leg supine twist variation is appropriate here because it's easy to execute. We offer you a number of other effective twists in Chapter 12.

If you're having a disc-related problem, be very careful of twists. If you have any negative symptoms, such as pain or numbness, leave the twist out and speak to your physician before adding it back to your program.

1. **Lie on your back with your knees bent and feet on the floor at hip width; extend your arms out from your sides like a *T,* with your palms down and in line with the top of your shoulders.**

2. **As you exhale, cross your right leg over your**

left leg, slowly lower your bent legs to the left side and then turn your head to the right as shown in Figure 22-17.

Keep your head on the floor.

3. As you inhale, bring your bent knees back up to the middle; as you exhale, slowly lower them back down to the same side.

4. Repeat Steps 1 through 3 three times and then stay down on the left side for 4 to 6 breaths.

5. Repeat Steps 1 through 4 with the left leg on top to the right side.

TIP If the cross-over twist variation is too difficult, try this same twist with the legs uncrossed and both feet on the ground.

Figure 22-17:
Bent-leg
supine twist.

Knees-to-chest posture: Apanasana

One of the rules of sequencing (which we cover in Chapter 15) is to always follow a twist with some kind of forward bend. Knees-to-chest is a classic forward bend to use when the posture preceding it is a floor twist, as in this back routine.

1. **Lie on your back and bend your knees in toward your chest.**

2. **Hold your shins just below your knees (see Figure 22-18a).**

3. **As you exhale, draw your knees inward, closer to your chest as demonstrated in Figure 22-18b.**

4. **Repeat Steps 2 and 3 three to four times and then relax and breathe, holding your shins for 6 to 8 breaths.**

If you have any knee problems, hold the backs of your thighs instead.

Figure 22-18:
Knees-to-chest posture.

Corpse posture with bent legs, repeated

When you come to the end of our back routine, the corpse posture variation we discuss at the beginning of the routine gives you a stable position to focus on your breathing and deeply relax your back. You don't want to skip this part. Stay in this posture for 25 to 30 breaths, making your exhalation slightly longer than your inhalation.

Covering your eyes can give a deeper relaxation effect. Use an eye bag or a scarf to cover your eyes to see whether you like it. (You can read more on eye bags and other props in Chapter 19.) Placing your feet comfortably up on a chair or a bed also adds a very calming effect and improves the circulation in your legs. It can even help improve your sleep.

Yoga Rx for Upper Backs and Necks

If you experience discomfort or limited movement in your upper back or neck, chances are your posture and possibly stress are contributing to the situation. This section helps you avoid those problems and gives you an upper back-friendly Yoga routine.

Do's and don'ts

The following list gives you some tips on what you can usually do to help your upper back and neck issues:

- ✔ Aim to perfect your mountain posture (see Chapter 7) and apply those lessons to your posture off the mat in your daily life.

- ✔ Discover how to let go of your tension with the relaxation techniques in Chapter 4. Becoming a student of Chapter 5's yogic breathing can also help you let go.

- ✔ Use the routine in the following section. You can also find DVD resources in the appendix.

Some actions can exacerbate your problems. Here are some things to avoid:

- ✔ No matter how much you may want to look like the models in many Yoga magazines, the headstand or full shoulder stand isn't for you. You can safely explore a world full of other postures.

- ✔ Avoid any neck routines that recommend full circles of the neck. This movement can cause serious problems, especially if you have a history of neck problems.

Upper back routine

This routine isn't for anyone in acute pain, and we don't recommend it for people experiencing numbness, tingling, or weakness in their neck, shoulders, or arms.

Seated chair posture

This posture is the base for the entire upper back routine, so make sure you understand how to sit in a way that feels steady and comfortable.

1. **Sit comfortably in an armless chair with your back up nice and tall; place your palms comfortably on your thighs.**

2. **Look straight ahead and bring your head comfortably back until the middle of your ears, your shoulders, and your hip sockets are in alignment as shown in Figure 22-19.**

3. **With your eyes open or closed, stay for six to eight breaths.**

Figure 22-19: Seated chair posture.

If your feet don't touch the floor, place a folded blanket, rolled-up mat, or other prop underneath them. Flip to Chapter 19 for more on using Yoga props.

Seated alternate arm raise sequence

Many of the muscles that go to your neck start between your shoulders, so this sequence is a good way to bring circulation to that area. Be sure to use both parts of the sequence, the arm raise and then the arm raise and head turn, to get the proper results.

1. **Start in the seated chair posture.**

2. **As you inhale, raise your slightly bent right arm as Figure 22-20a illustrates.**

3. **As you exhale, return your right palm to your right thigh; repeat Steps 2 and 3, alternating with your right and left arms two to three times each.**

4. **Continue raising and alternating your arms and turning your head away from each arm for two to three additional rounds as in Figure 22-20b.**

Figure 22-20:
Seated
alternate
arm raise
sequence.

Seated shoulder rolls

The neck and shoulders are one of the most frequent sites of tension for Westerners. Seated shoulder rolls can bring instant stress relief to stored-up tension.

1. **Start in the seated chair posture.**

2. **Hang your arms at your sides and roll your shoulders up and back as you inhale (see Figure 22-21).**

3. **As you exhale, roll your shoulders down.**

4. **Repeat Steps 2 and 3 four to six times and then reverse the direction of the rolls for four to six repetitions.**

Figure 22-21: *Seated shoulder rolls.*

Wing-and-prayer sequence

Think of your upper back and neck as your wingspan; this sequence (as well as those in the following sections) helps you keep that wingspan in balance.

1. **Start in the seated chair posture.**

2. **Join your palms together in the prayer position**

512

as in Figure 22-22a.

3. As you inhale, raise your arms comfortably above your head, keeping your hands in the prayer position as Figure 22-22b demonstrates.

4. As you exhale, bring your hands and arms back down, still maintaining prayer position.

5. As you inhale, separate your hands and move your arms out like wings to the sides at about shoulder height, lifting your chest and looking straight ahead as illustrated in Figure 22-22c.

6. As you exhale, bring your hands and arms to the starting position in Step 2.

7. Repeat Steps 1 through 6 four to six times.

Figure 22-22:
Wing-and-prayer sequence.

Mirror-on-the-hand sequence

This sequence safely reaches very subtle muscles in your neck and shoulders.

1. Start in the seated chair posture.

2. As you inhale, raise the back of your right hand

to eye level as shown in **Figure 22-23a.**

3. **As you exhale, bring your right hand inward and place your palm and fingers at the top of your left shoulder, turning your eyes and head down and to the left as you follow your right hand as Figure 22-23b illustrates.**

   If you have a problem rotating your neck outward to the right or the left, only turn as far as you feel comfortable.

4. **As you inhale, return the back of your right hand to eye level and keep it moving and opening around to the right as far as is comfortable (see Figure 22-23c).**

5. **As you exhale, bring the back of the right hand in front of you again at eye level.**

6. **Continue exhaling as you bring the right hand back down to the seated chair posture.**

7. **Repeat Steps 1 through 6, alternating right and left sides three to four times each.**

Figure 22-23:
Mirror-on-
the-hand
sequence.

Newspaper sequence

This is the most challenging sequence to coordinate. Give yourself some time to get used to it, and it may become one of your favorites.

1. **Start in the seated chair posture.**

2. **Inhale and then, as you exhale, move both hands up to eye level with your palms facing you as though you were looking at a newspaper (Figure 22-24a demonstrates).**

3. **As you inhale, move both hands up and follow your hands with your eyes and head until your hands are just above your forehead as shown in Figure 22-24b.**

   Try not to turn your head too far back when you're looking up at your hands. Think of rotating up from the level of your ears rather than your collar.

4. **As you exhale, bring your chin down to your chest without moving your arms as in Figure 22-24c.**

5. **As you inhale, separate your hands and move your arms out like wings to the sides at about shoulder height, lifting your chest and looking straight ahead as illustrated in Figure 22-24d.**

6. **As you exhale, extend your bent arms forward like they're going over a log and round your back like a camel as you look down (see Figure 22-24e).**

7. **As you inhale, lift your chest; rotate your elbows and palms inward as you raise your**

hands back to eye level as in Step 2 (see Figure 22-24a).

8. **Repeat Steps 1 through 7 four to six times.**

Figure 22-24:
The newspaper sequence.

Seated sage twist

This twist rejuvenates the upper back as well as the entire spine. It also tones the abdomen.

Resist the temptation to crank this twist too hard. Move slowly and carefully. If you experience pain or discomfort, leave the twist out of your routine and check with your health professional before further use.

1. **Start in the seated chair posture turned sideways with the back of the chair to your right; hold the sides of the chair back with your hands as Figure 22-25 illustrates.**

2. **As you inhale, extend or lift your spine and head upward.**

3. As you exhale, twist your torso and head farther to the right.

4. Repeat Steps 2 and 3, gradually twisting to your comfort level, and then stay in the twist for four to six breaths.

5. Repeat Steps 1 through 4 on the left side.

Figure 22-25: Seated sage twist.

Seated forward bend variation

A twist is almost always followed by a forward bend to rebalance the spine and hips, so here's one to counter the twist in the preceding section.

1. Start in the seated chair posture turned sideways with the chair back on either your left or right.

2. As you exhale, bend forward from the hips and slide your hands down your legs as you hang your head, chest, and arms comfortably as shown in Figure 22-26.

3. Stay in Step 2 for six to eight breaths.

Figure 22-26:
Seated forward bend variation.

Seated neck and shoulder massage

This simple technique is very good for releasing land mines between your neck and shoulders.

Holding, squeezing, or compressing tight spots is called *ischemic massage* and is often used by body workers to release trigger points or sensitive and irritable areas of the body.

1. **Start in the seated chair posture and bring your right arm up and across toward your left shoulder; place your right palm down between the top of your left shoulder and your neck as illustrated in Figure 22-27.**

2. **Slowly and gently massage the surface area between the neck and the left shoulder in a circular motion (starting toward the neck) six to eight times, noticing any tight spots.**

3. **Find the tightest spots you identified in Step 2 and grab or squeeze each one firmly for six to eight counts.**

518

4. Finish the self-massage by repeating Step 2 six to eight times.

5. Repeat Steps 1 through 4 with the left hand on your right side.

Figure 22-27:
Seated neck and shoulder massage.

Seated relaxation

All of the concentration, breath, and movement leads to this moment. You may also replace this breathing exercise with any of the relaxation techniques in Chapter 4.

1. Start in the seated chair posture with your eyes closed as in Figure 22-28.

2. Use belly breathing (see Chapter 5) and gradually increase the length of your exhalation until you reach your comfortable maximum.

3. Take 20 to 30 belly breaths at your comfortable maximum and then gradually come back to your normal resting breath.

Figure 22-28:
Seated relaxation.

Part V

The Part of Tens

The 5th Wave   By Rich Tennant

"Oh, how wonderful! A CD to play during my Yoga workouts! 'Sweatin' With The Maharishi'."

In this part . . .

This part is the place to turn if you want to get clear about why you're practicing or ought to be practicing Yoga, or about how to approach Yoga correctly. It's full of fun little snippets of information that remind you how wonderful Yoga practice is. We also we give you the top places in the United States and Canada to contact in case you're thinking of enrolling in a Yoga class or workshop to get started.

Chapter 23

Ten Tips for a Great Yoga Practice

....

In This Chapter

▶ Preparing yourself for proper practice
▶ Creating an engaging and supportive environment

....

To succeed at anything, you must know two things: the ground rules and yourself. In this chapter, we give you ten hot tips for growing your Yoga practice into a sturdy, fruit-laden tree. If you bear these points in mind, you can expect to reap the benefits of your efforts surprisingly quickly. Although we don't promise overnight miracles, we're confident that regular, correct Yoga practice can bring you multiple advantages — physically, mentally, and spiritually.

Understand Yoga

To engage in Yoga successfully, you must first understand what it is and how it works. Sometimes people rush into Yoga practice without knowing anything about it, and then they have to work through a bunch of misconceptions before they can benefit from it.

 This book gives you a basic understanding of the nature and principles of this age-old discipline — enough for a solid start. But make time to read other books on Yoga to deepen your comprehension (see the appendix for suggestions on resources).

Traditional Yoga involves study, a key aspect of practice for thousands of years. We especially recommend that you acquaint yourself with the actual literature of Yoga — notably the *Yoga-Sutra* of Patanjali and the *Bhagavad-Gita* — through the many translations available today. The Yoga tradition is vast and highly diverse. Discover which approach speaks to you the most.

Be Clear (and Realistic) about Your Goals and Needs

If you want your Yoga practice to be successful, take the time to consider your personal situation carefully and then set your goals based on your abilities and needs. Ask yourself, "How much free time do I have or want to make available for Yoga? What are my expectations? Do I want to become or stay fit and trim? Do I want to be able to relax more and discover the art of meditation? Do I want to adopt Yoga as a lifestyle or explore the spiritual dimension of life?" When you're realistic, you're less likely to experience disappointment or guilt when your schedule seems overwhelming.

 If you're dealing with health issues or physical impediments, make sure that you consult your physician before you launch your Yoga practice.

Commit Yourself to Growth

Even if you don't choose to practice Yoga as a lifestyle, keep an open mind about Yoga's involvement in your life. Allow it to transform not only your body but also your mind. Don't put a ceiling on your own development or assume that you're incapable of ever achieving a certain Yoga posture or learning how to meditate. Let Yoga gently work with your physical and mental limitations and expand your abilities and help you outgrow useless attitudes and negative thoughts and discover new horizons.

Stay for the Long Haul

Spoiled by their consumerist societies, most people expect quick fixes. Although Yoga can work miracles in a short span of time, it's not like instant coffee. To derive the full benefits from Yoga, you have to apply yourself diligently, which also nicely strengthens your character. The longer you practice Yoga, the more enjoyable and beneficial it becomes. Give Yoga at least a year to prove itself to you. We promise you won't be disappointed. In fact, you may very well come out of that year with a lifelong commitment to growing with Yoga!

Develop Good Habits from the Beginning

Bad habits die hard, so cultivate good Yoga habits from the outset. If possible, take two or three lessons from a qualified Yoga teacher, either in a group class or privately. At least read our book — and other practical Yoga books — carefully before trying out the postures and breathing exercises.

Wrong practice can do damage! Protect yourself by proceeding slowly and following the instructions step by step. Err on the cautious side. If in doubt, always consult a teacher or knowledgeable practitioner.

Vary Your Routine to Avoid Boredom

After you enjoy the initial wash of enthusiasm, your mind may start playing tricks on you. (Here are some favorite expressions of doubt: "Maybe Yoga doesn't work." "It doesn't work for *me*." "I really have other more important things to do." "I don't feel like practicing today.") If you're easily bored, vary your program periodically to keep your interest alive. Slogging through Yoga or any exercise program serves no purpose. Cultivate what the Zen Buddhists call "beginner's mind": Approach your Yoga sessions (and, in fact, everything else) with the same intensity and freshness that you brought to your very first session. If you focus on each exercise properly, your mind doesn't have time to feel bored. Also, the more you involve yourself in the spirit of Yoga, the more centered you become, lessening your likelihood of needing an exercise potpourri.

 Yoga For Dummies, 2nd Edition, gives you a well-tested formula for creating many efficient routines for a variety of situations. You can make your programs as diversified and challenging as you like. Check out Chapter 15.

Make Awareness and Breath Your Allies

Yoga practice is so potent because, if you practice it correctly, it combines physical movement with awareness and proper breathing. Awareness and breath are Yoga's secret weapons. The sooner you catch on to this concept, the more quickly you can enjoy really satisfying results. Bringing awareness to your exercise routine also automatically strengthens your overall capacity for concentration and mindfulness (which we cover in Chapter 21). You're able to work more efficiently and better appreciate your leisure time. In particular, conscious breathing during the exercises greatly enhances the effects of your practice on your body and mind, equipping you with the vitality you need to meet the challenges of a busy life.

Do Your Best and Don't Worry about the Rest

People often anxiously watch their progress. Progress isn't linear; sometimes you seem to take a step back, only to take a big leap forward in due course. Be diligent but relaxed about your Yoga practice. Perfectionism serves no purpose other than to frustrate you and irritate others. In aspiring to reach your goal, be kind to yourself (and others). Don't worry about what may or may not happen down the line. Focus on practicing now and leave the rest to the power of Yoga, providence, and your good karma (see Chapter 1).

Allow Your Body to Speak Up

Your body is your best friend and counselor, and listening to it is an art well worth cultivating. If something doesn't feel right, it probably isn't. Trust your bodily instincts and intuitions not only in your Yoga practice but also in daily life. All too frequently, your body tells you one thing and your mind another. Learn to go with your body.

When practicing Hatha Yoga, be especially careful about letting your desire to achieve quick results get in the way of common sense and bodily wisdom. For instance, if a forward or backward bend feels risky, don't test your luck. Or if your body tells you that you aren't ready for the head-stand (which we don't recommend for beginners anyway), don't fall victim to your own ambition.

Share Yoga

In the beginning, plan to practice Yoga with others until you find your own momentum. Sometimes everyone needs a little encouragement, and a supportive environment is a great bonus. If you don't go to a regular Yoga class, take the initiative to enlist an interested family member or friend in your Yoga practice. Make sure, however, that you keep any missionary zeal under wraps. Yoga is a wonderful gift to give to anyone, and so offer it in an attractive way: with love and tempered enthusiasm.

Chapter 24

Ten Good Reasons to Practice Yoga

Your journey of discovery in the world of Yoga is not only exciting but also immensely rewarding. In this chapter, we give you ten excellent reasons to begin that journey now and persist in it.

The effects of regular Yoga practice are pervasive and astonishing, and you can see good results very quickly. If you practice Hatha Yoga (the form of Yoga that deals specifically with the body), you may first notice an improvement in your flexibility, muscle tone, and overall fitness. Certainly, expect to feel better. Other wonderful benefits manifest as you continue to practice regularly and go deeper into Yoga. You have every reason to proceed with confidence!

Yoga Helps You Maintain, Recover, or Improve Your Health

Yoga is an amazing stress-buster. When you consider that 75 to 90 percent of all visits to the doctor are related to stress, Yoga's holistic approach is a prudent first choice for fostering well-being. Through its relaxation, postural, breathing, and meditation exercises as well as dietary rules, Yoga can effectively lower your level of tension and anxiety. Thus, yogic practice boosts your immune system, which helps keep illness at bay and facilitates the physical healing process if you're already sick. Research demonstrates that Yoga is a very effective way of dealing with a variety of health problems from hypertension, adult-onset diabetes, and respiratory illnesses (such as asthma) to sleep disturbance, chronic headache, and lower back pain. Yoga can help improve your cardiovascular functions, digestion, and eyesight and even enable you to control pain. You can practice Yoga as both remedial and preventive medicine. You can't find a cheaper health and life insurance policy! Moreover, Yoga is pain-free. In fact, Yoga helps overcome all forms of suffering (see Chapter 20).

Yoga Makes You Fit and Energetic

Yoga relaxes your body and mind, thereby enabling you to mobilize all the energy you need in order to deal efficiently with the many challenges at home and at work. Yoga can greatly promote your body's flexibility, fitness, strength, and stamina. In addition, Yoga may even help you shed surplus pounds.

Yoga Balances Your Mind

Yoga not only assists you in maintaining or recovering your physical well-being (see the earlier section "Yoga Helps You Maintain, Recover, or Improve Your Health") but also has a profound influence on your mind. The mind is the source of many of your troubles — sooner or later, the body reflects wrong attitudes, negative thoughts, and emotional imbalance that your mind holds. Yoga is a powerful tool for clearing your mind and freeing you from mood swings. Yogic practice supports greater results than any tranquilizer and without the undesirable side effects of drugs. It balances you without dulling your mind. Through Yoga, you can stay alert but relaxed.

Yoga Is a Powerful Aid for Personal Growth

Yoga can help you discover the body's hidden potential. Your body is a marvelous instrument, but you need to play it properly to produce beautiful, harmonious melodies. Yoga also can guide you safely into the exploration of the hidden aspects of the mind, especially higher states of consciousness (such as ecstasy and enlightenment, which we explain in Chapter 21). It progressively peels away misconceptions about yourself and about life in general and reveals your true nature, which is uncomplicated and blissful.

Yoga Is Truly Comprehensive and Empowering

Yoga offers you a sensible, growth-oriented lifestyle that

covers all aspects of life from cradle to grave. Its repertoire includes techniques for optimal physical and mental health, for dealing creatively with the challenges of modern life, for transforming your sexual life, and even for making creative use of your dream life through the art of lucid dreaming (discussed in Chapter 20). Yoga makes you feel comfortable with your body, improves your self-image and self-esteem, and enhances your power of concentration and memory. Ultimately, Yoga empowers you to discover your spiritual essence and to live free from fear and other limiting emotions and thoughts.

Yoga Helps You Harmonize Your Social Relationships

By giving you a new outlook on life, Yoga can help you improve your relationships with family, friends, co-workers, and others. It gives you the means to develop patience, tolerance, compassion, and forgiveness. Through the techniques of Yoga, you can gain control of your mind and liberate yourself from obsessions and undesirable habits, which can stand in the way of satisfying relationships. Yoga also shows you how to live at peace with the world and attuned to your essential nature, the spirit or Self. It provides you with all you need to harmonize and beautify your life.

Yoga Enhances Your Awareness

Yoga enables you to greatly intensify your awareness, as we discuss in Chapter 1. Thus, yogic practice empowers you to approach all life situations, even crises, with clarity and serenity. In addition, Yoga makes you more sensitive to your bodily rhythms, heightens your five senses, and even develops your intuitive faculty (the so-called sixth sense). Most significantly, Yoga puts you in touch with the spiritual reality that is the source of your everyday mind and awareness.

Yoga Combines Well with Other Disciplines

Although Yoga is complete in itself, you can easily combine it with any kind of sports or physical workout, including aerobics and weightlifting. You also can practice Yoga in conjunction with any existing mental discipline, including mnemonics (memorization) and chess. Not only is Yoga compatible in all cases, but it's also bound to improve your performance.

Yoga Is Easy and Convenient

Yoga doesn't require you to work up a sweat (unless you're practicing some modern aerobic-type Yoga). You can always look pretty cool! You can practice Yoga in the comfort of your own home — or, in fact, anywhere. Although you don't need to spend time traveling from place to place, beginners in particular should consider joining a Yoga class — even your trip there and back offers opportunities for a Yoga experience. Yoga creates rather than consumes time — a major benefit in the busy and stressed lives of Westerners!

Yoga Is Liberating

Yoga can put you more in touch with your true nature, giving you a sense of fulfillment, inner worth, and confidence.

By assisting you in reducing egotism and negative thoughts and emotions, Yoga has the power to bring you closer to lasting happiness. It builds your willpower and puts you in charge of your own life.

Appendix

Additional Yoga Resources

Here are some Yoga resources we couldn't get into the rest of the book. Hopefully, the variety of media we offer here helps you take that next step on your Yoga journey.

Discovering Yoga Organizations

In Chapter 24, we give you our choices for the top ten Yoga centers in the United States and Canada. Here are a few additional names and addresses to help you with your explorations.

✔ **International Association of Yoga Therapists:** Founded in 1979 by Larry Payne, PhD, and Richard Miller, PhD, and now directed by John Kepner, this association has over 2,500 members, publishes an annual journal and a triannual publication (see the "Peeking into Periodicals" section later in this appendix), and conducts an annual conference. Its Web site provides a wealth of scholarly materials on the therapeutic use of Yoga. You can find it at International Association of Yoga Therapists, PO

Box 12890, Prescott, AZ 86304; phone 928-541-0182; Web site www.iayt.org.

✔ **Gary Kraftsow American Viniyoga Institute:** The institute, directed by Gary and Mirka Kraftsow, offers classes and personal sessions as well as retreats and training programs in Yoga therapy in the Viniyoga style. Check it out at Gary Kraftsow American Viniyoga Institute, LLC, Oakland, CA; phone 808-572-1414; e-mail info@viniyoga.com, Web site www.viniyoga.com.

✔ **Phoenix Rising Yoga Therapy:** Founded and directed by Michael Lee, this program offers a range of classes and workshops, as well as teacher training. (Head to the following section for more teacher training recommendations.) You can find more information at The Phoenix Rising Center, 5 Mountain Street, PO Box 200, Bristol, VT 05443; phone 800-288-9642; e-mail info@pryt.com, Web site www.pryt.com/.

✔ **Yoga Therapy Rx at Loyola Marymount University:** Coauthor Larry founded and directs this program, which offers three-year training programs in Yoga therapy and integrative medicine. Check it out at LMU Extension Programs, One LMU Drive, Los Angeles, CA 90045; phone 310-338-2358; Web-site www.lmu.edu/academics/extension/crs/certificates/yoga_rx.htm.

Taking a Look at Teacher Training and Academic Programs

In addition to the teacher training programs listed in

Chapter 24, we recommend that you check out the following organizations if you're interested in becoming a Yoga teacher:

✔ **American Sanskrit Institute:** The institute, directed by Vyaas Houston, offers extensive courses (including immersion training) in the Sanskrit language and also has CDs available for study. Find out more at American Sanskrit Institute, 980 Ridge Road, Brick, NJ 08724; phone 800-459-4176 or 732-840-4104; e-mail vyaas.houston@gmail.com, Web site www.americansanskrit.com.

✔ **American Institute of Vedic Studies:** This organization offers in-depth correspondence courses on teaching Yoga, Vedas, and Ayurveda. It's directed by Dr. David Frawley (Vamadeva Shastri), and you can contact it at American Institute of Vedic Studies, PO Box 8357, Santa Fe, NM 87504; phone 505-983-9385; e-mail vedicinst@aol.com, Web site www.vedanet.com.

✔ **International Yoga Studies:** Founded and directed by Sandra Summerfield Kozak, this program offers a well-rounded teacher training program based on the standards developed by the European Union of Yoga. Check it out at International Yoga Studies, 692 Andrew Court, Benicia, CA 94510; phone 707-745-5224; e-mail iysusa@internationalyogastudies.com, Web site www. internationalyogastudies.com/.

✔ **Integrative Yoga Therapy:** This organization, founded and directed by Joseph LePage, consists of a professional training program bridging the insights of Yoga and the latest advances in mind-body healing. IYT also offers advanced and continuing training for its graduates. You can find it at Integrative Yoga Therapy, 5345 Darrow Rd. #4, Hudson, OH 44236; phone 800-750-9642 or 415-670-9642; e-mail info@iytyogatherapy.com, Web site www.iytyogatherapy.com/.

✔ **Traditional Yoga Studies:** Founded by Brenda Feuerstein in Canada, this study program offers several substantial distance-learning programs on Yoga philosophy and history designed and tutored by coauthor Georg, a Yoga philosophy and history teacher Training Manual, and several books and recordings. Find out more at Traditional Yoga Studies, PO Box 661, Eastend, Saskatchewan, S0N 0T0, Canada; e-mail tyslearning@sasktel.net, Web site www.traditionalyogastudies.com/.

✔ **Yoga Ed:** This organization develops and produces trainings and products for teachers, parents, children, and health professionals that improve academic achievement, physical fitness, emotional intelligence and stress management. It also offers health and wellness programs. Get more info by calling 310-471-1742 or going online at www.yogaed.com.

Knowing Other Significant Organizations in the U.S. and Canada

Check out these great establishments:

✔ **The Hard and The Soft Yoga Institute:** Directed by Beryl Bender Birch, the institute offers *Power Yoga* — an athletic and precision approach to Hatha Yoga. Find out more at The Hard and The Soft

Yoga Institute, PO Box 5009, East Hampton, NY 11937; phone 631-324-8409; e-mail info@power-yoga.com, Web site www.power-yoga.com/.

- **Moksha Yoga:** Founded by Ted Grand and Jessica Robertson, this group of independent *Hot Yoga* studios (Yoga practiced in particularly warm rooms) is committed to ethical, compassionate and environmentally conscious living. You can find it at 68 Hogarth Avenue, Toronto, Ontario, M4K 1K3, Canada; phone 416-778-9898; e-mail info@ mokshayoga.ca, Web site http://www.mokshayoga.ca/.

- **The Movement Center:** This organization operates a full-service Yoga center and is one of the larger independent publishers of Yoga-related books, tapes, and videos in the United States. It's directed by Swami Chetanananda, and you can get more information at The Movement Center, PO Box 13310, Portland, OR 97232; phone 503-231-0383, fax 1-503-236-9878; e-mail info@themovementcenter. com, Web site themovementcenter.com/index.php.

- **White Lotus Foundation:** Established in 1967 and codirected by Ganga White and Tracey Rich, the foundation offers a synthesis of classical and contemporary styles of Yoga as well as teacher training programs and retreats. Check it out at White Lotus Foundation, 2500 San Marcos Pass, Santa Barbara, CA 93105; phone 805-964-1944, fax 1-805-964-9617; e-mail info@whitelotus.org, Web site www.whitelotus.org/.

Mapping Major Overseas Organizations

Here we bring you a selection of leading Yoga organizations outside the United States; these sources can refer you to teachers during your overseas travels.

Europe

The following list gives you some of the top European Yoga organizations:

- **The British Wheel of Yoga:** Founded in 1965, this program has around 4,000 Yoga teachers as members and publishes *Spectrum* magazine (see "Peeking into Periodicals" later in this appendix). Check it out at The British Wheel of Yoga, 25 Jermyn Street, Sleaford, Lincolnshire, NG34 7RU; phone 01529-306851, fax 01529-303233; e-mail office@bwy.org.uk, Web site www.bwy.org.uk/.

- **Life Foundation:** This large, full-service Yoga and humanitarian organization founded by Dr. Manushkh Patel is dedicated to *Dru Yoga* (a mix of teachings based on ancient Yoga principals) through international peace walks, a cancer center, and therapeutics. It also maintains a large selection of books, audios, and videos. Get more information at Life Foundation Course Centre, Nant Francon, Bangor, North Wales, LL57 3LX, UK; phone 44-(0)1248-602900, fax 44-(0)1248-602004; e-mail enquiries@lifefoundation.org.uk, Web site www.lifefoundation.com/.

- **Weg Der Mitte:** Founded by Daya Mullins, PhD, this organization offers Yoga teacher and holistic practitioner certification courses. It's located in Berlin, with a retreat center in Gerode, Germany. Check it out at Weg Der Mitte, Ahornstrasse 18, D-14163, Berlin, Germany; phone 011-49-30-

813-1040, fax 011-49-30-813-8281; e-mail berlin@
wegdermitte.de; Web site www.wegdermitte.de.

Latin America

Take a look at these Latin American Yoga havens:

- ✔ **Indra Devi Foundation:** Founded by David Lifar,
  this Argentine program is the largest Hatha Yoga
  center in South America, with over 2,000 students
  per week in three locations. It has a newsletter and
  teacher training programs. Find more at Indra Devi
  Foundation, Azuenaga 762, Buenos Aires, Argentina
  1029; e-mail contactenos@fundacion-indra-devi.org,
  Web site fundacion-indra-devi.org/.

- ✔ **Latin American Union of Yoga:** This union,
  founded in 1985, organizes annual Yoga conferences
  and in particular promotes artistic and Olympic
  Yoga sports. It also publishes the magazine
  Yoga Integral. You can get more information at
  Latin American Union of Yoga, Calle Piedras
  3364 esq. Rivera, Fray Bentos (Río Negro),
  Uruguay; phone 00598-562-3340; e-mail info@
  unionlatinoamericanadeyoga.org, Web site www.
  unionlatinoamericanadeyoga.org/.

Australia and New Zealand

The International Yoga Teachers Association, directed
by Susan Kirkham, has a membership of several hundred
Yoga teachers in New Zealand and Australia and offers
teacher training courses. It also publishes a newsletter for
members. Get more info at IYTA, GPO Box 1380, Syd-
ney NSW 2001, Australia; phone 61-2-9489-9851; e-mail
info@iyta.org.au, Web site www.iyta.org.au/.

India

- **Bihar School of Yoga:** Founded in 1963 and today directed by Swami Niranjanananda Sarasvati, this school is known for its high standards of teacher training and advanced programs, especially in Kriya Yoga and Kundalini Yoga. It also has a Yoga university. For more information, contact The Registrar, Bihar Yoga Bharati, Ganga Darshan, Fort, Munger, Bihar 811201, India; phone 91-(0)-6344-222430, fax 91-(0)-344-220169; Web site www. yogavision.net/.

- **Gitananda Ashram:** Established by the late Dr. Swami Gitananda Giri and presently headed by Meenakshi Devi, this very active school offers many programs, including a correspondence course, and the monthly magazine *Yoga Life* (see the "Peeking into Periodicals" section later in this appendix). Check it out at Gitananda Ashram, 16A Mettu Street, Chinnamudaliarchavady, Kottukuppam (Via Pondicherry) 605 104 Tamil Nadu, India; Web site www.icyer.com/.

- **Krishnamacharya Yoga Mandiram:** This nonprofit institute founded by T.K.V Desikachar (the son of T. Krishnamacharya) is based in India and dedicated to spreading the teachings of T. Krishnamacharya with his holistic and secular approach of adapting Yoga to the individual's needs. Its training and Yoga therapy programs are open to international students, and its Web site offers a weekly sutra, asana, and "answer from the expert" as well as a bookstore. Find more info at Krishnamacharya Yoga Mandiram, New No.31 (Old

#13) Fourth Cross Street, R K Nagar, Chennai -
600 028, India; phone 91-44-24937998/24933092;
e-mail admin@kym.org, Web site www.kym.org/.

- **Ramamani Iyengar Memorial Yoga Institute:**
Founded and directed by B.K.S. Iyengar, the
institute is the hub of the world's most widespread
style of Hatha Yoga — Iyengar Yoga (head to
Chapter 1 for more info). The Institute has trained
thousands of Yoga teachers. Get more information
at Ramamani Iyengar Memorial Yoga Institute
(RIMYI), 1107 B/1 Hare Krishna Mandir Road,
Model Colony, Shivaji Nagar, Pune 411 016,
Maharashtra, India; phone 91-20-2565-6134; e-mail
info@bksiyengar.com, Web site www.bksiyengar.com/.

Tapping Into Yoga Props

Chapter 19 covers using props in your Yoga practice. Here
we give you some resources to help acquaint you with the
possibilities. The publication *Yoga Journal* is another excellent source for companies specializing in Yoga paraphernalia,
such as mats, blocks, straps, outfits, and so on.

- Yoga Props, 3055 23rd Street, San Francisco, CA
94110; phone 888-856-YOGA (9642) or 415-285-
YOGA (9642), fax 1-415-920-YOGA (9642); e-mail
service@yogaprops.net, Web site www.yogaprops.net/.

- Hugger Mugger, 1190 S Pioneer Rd, Salt Lake City,
UT 84104; phone 800-473-4888; e-mail comments@
huggermugger.com, Web site www.huggermugger.
com/.

Checking Out Top-Notch Web Sites

Yoga's presence on the Internet is growing rapidly, so here are some excellent sites for you to visit. Most of them contain links to other sites.

- ✔ **Hindu Tantrik Homepage (www.shivashakti. com/):** A fine Tantra site maintained by Michael Magee, translator of several Sanskrit texts

- ✔ **Samata International (www.samata.com/):** Source for coauthor Larry's DVDs and books and information about his courses, classes, and retreats, including Yoga Rx and Prime of Life Yoga

- ✔ **Traditional Yoga Studies (www. traditionalyogastudies.com/):** Web site featuring writings by coauthor Georg

- ✔ **Yoga Minded (www.yogaminded.com):** Offers Yoga education materials for teens

- ✔ **Yoga Playgrounds (yogaplaygrounds.ning.com/):** Offers Yoga resources for teaching Yoga to children for classroom teachers, yoga teachers, parents, and teachers of children with special needs

Lingering at the Yoga Library

The following resources are among the better books available today on Yoga and Yoga-related topics. They represent a small selection from a huge body of literature. If you have Internet access, check out the long list of Yoga books available on www.amazon.com.

Reference works and general introductions

- *The Shambhala Encyclopedia of Yoga* by Georg Feuerstein (Shambhala Publications)

- *The Yoga Tradition: Its History, Literature, Philosophy, and Practice,* 3rd Edition, by Georg Feuerstein (Hohm Press)

- *The Shambhala Guide to Yoga* by Georg Feuerstein (Shambhala Publications)

- *The Tree of Yoga* by B.K.S. Iyengar (Shambhala Publications)

Hatha Yoga (beginners and advanced)

- *The Deeper Dimensions of Yoga* by Georg Feuerstein (Shambhala Publications)

- *Hatha Yoga: The Hidden Language* by Swami Sivananda Radha (Timeless Books)

- *The Heart of Yoga: Developing a Personal Practice* by T.K.V. Desikachar (Inner Traditions)

- *Light on Pranayama: The Yogic Art of Breathing* by B.K.S. Iyengar (Crossroad)

- *Light on Yoga* by B.K.S. Iyengar (Schocken Books)

- *The Awakened Union of Breath, Body and Mind* by Frank Jude Boccio (Shambhala Publications)

- *The New Yoga for People Over 50* by Suza Francina (Health Communications)

- *Power Yoga: The Total Strength and Flexibility Workout* by Beryl Bender Birch (Fireside Books)

545

✔ *Relax and Renew: Restful Yoga for Stressful Times* by Judith Lasater (Rodmell Press)

✔ *A Systematic Course in the Ancient Tantric Techniques of Yoga and Kriya* by Swami Satyananda Saraswati (Bihar School of Yoga)

✔ *Yoga for Body, Breath, and Mind: A Guide to Personal Reintegration* by A. G. Mohan (Rudra Press)

✔ *Yoga: The Spirit and Practice of Moving Into Stillness* by Erich Schiffman (Pocket Books)

Raja (classical), Jnana, Bhakti, and Karma Yoga

✔ *The Essence of Yoga* by Bernard Bouanchaud (Rudra Press)

✔ *Raja-Yoga* by Swami Vivekananda (Ramakrishna-Vivekananda Center)

✔ *The Yoga-Sutra of Patanjali: A New Translation and Commentary* by Georg Feuerstein (Inner Traditions)

✔ *Jnana-Yoga* by Swami Vivekananda (Ramakrishna-Vivekananda Center)

✔ *Ramana Maharshi and the Path of Self-Knowledge* by Arthur Osborne

✔ *Karma-Yoga and Bhakti-Yoga* by Swami Vivekananda (Ramakrishna-Vivekananda Center)

✔ *The Yoga of Spiritual Devotion: A Modern Translation of the Narada Bhakti Sutras* by Prem Prakash (Inner Traditions International)

Tantra and Kundalini Yoga

- *Energies of Transformation: A Guide to the Kundalini Process* by Bonnie Greenwell (Shakti River Press)

- *Kundalini Yoga for the West* by Swami Sivananda Radha (Timeless Books)

- *Layayoga: An Advanced Method of Concentration* by Shyam Sundar Goswami (Inner Traditions International)

- *Living With Kundalini: The Autobiography of Gopi Krishna* edited by Leslie Shepard (Shambhala Publications)

- *The Serpent Power* by John Woodroffe (Ganesh & Co)

- *Tantra: The Path of Ecstasy* by Georg Feuerstein (Shambhala Publications)

Meditation, mantras, and prayer

- *Healing Words* by Larry Dossey (HarperSanFrancisco)

- *Mantra & Meditation* by Usharbudh Arya (Himalayan International Institute)

- *Meditation For Dummies*, 2nd Edition, by Stephan Bodian (Wiley)

Yoga for pregnancy and children

- *Bountiful, Beautiful, Blissful: Experience the Natural Power of Pregnancy and Birth with Kundalini Yoga and Meditation* by Gurmukh Kaur Khalsa (St. Martin's Press)

- *Yogakids: Educating the Whole Child Through Yoga* by Marsha Wenig

Yoga therapy

- *Phoenix Rising Yoga Therapy: A Bridge from Body to Soul* by Michael Lee (Health Communications)

- *Yoga as Medicine: The Yogic Prescription for Health and Healing* by Yoga Journal and Timothy McCall (Bantam Books)

- *Yoga for Common Ailments* by Robin Munro, R. Nagarathna, and H. R. Nagendra (Simon & Schuster)

- *Yoga RX: A Step-by-Step Program to Promote Health, Wellness, and Healing for Common Ailments* by Larry Payne and Richard Usatine (Broadway Books)

- *Yoga Therapy: A Guide to the Therapeutic Use of Yoga and Ayurveda for Health and Fitness* by A.G. Mohan and Indra Mohan (Shambhala)

General Yoga topics

- *The Art of Positive Feeling* by Swami Jyotirmayananda (Yoga Research Foundation)

- *Dancing with Siva: Hinduism's Contemporary Catechism* by Satguru Sivaya Subramuniyaswami (Himalayan Academy)

- *The Future of the Body: Explorations Into the Further Evolution of Human Nature* by Michael Murphy (Jeremy Tarcher)

- *Golden Rules for Everyday Life* by Omraam Mikhaël

Aïvanhov (Prosveta)

- ✔ *Green Dharma* by Georg Feuerstein and Brenda Feuerstein (Traditional Yoga Studies)

- ✔ *Green Yoga* by Georg Feuerstein and Brenda Feuerstein (Traditional Yoga Studies)

- ✔ *Health, Healing and Beyond: Yoga and the Living Tradition of Krishnamacharya* by T.K.V. Desikachar with R.H. Cravens (Aperture)

- ✔ *Lucid Dreaming* by Stephen LaBerge (Ballentine)

- ✔ *Lucid Waking: Mindfulness and the Spiritual Potential of Humanity* by Georg Feuerstein (Inner Traditions International)

- ✔ *The Nine Stages of Spiritual Apprenticeship: Understanding the Student-Teacher Relationship* by Greg Bogart (Dawn Mountain Press)

- ✔ *The Relaxation Response* by Herbert Benson (Avon Books)

- ✔ *The Tibetan Book of Living and Dying* by Sogyal Rinpoche (HarperSanFrancisco)

- ✔ *A Year to Live: How to Live this Year As If It Were Your Last* by Stephen Levine (Bell Tower)

- ✔ *Yoga Morality* by Georg Feuerstein (Hohm Press)

Peeking into Periodicals

Although periodicals aren't exactly environmentally friendly, we provide information for the better-known periodicals that cover Yoga from various points of view. Just be sure to recycle them when you're done.

- *Hinduism Today:* A monthly magazine for students of Yoga and Hinduism. Offers a free online version and a paid hardcopy, print-edition subscription. Find out more at Hinduism Today, 107 Kaholalele Road, Kapaa, HI 96746; Web site www.hinduismtoday.com/.

- *International Journal of Yoga Therapy* (formerly *Journal of the International Association of Yoga Therapists*): An annual journal for professionals interested in the restorative applications of Yoga and a triannual publication entitled *Yoga Therapy Today.* Check it out at International Association of Yoga Therapists, 115 S. McCormick, Suite 3, Prescott, AZ 86304; phone 928-541-0004; Web site www.iayt. org/.

- *Yoga & Health:* A monthly Yoga magazine. You can find it at Yoga Today Ltd., PO Box 2130, Seaford, Sussex BN25 9BF, United Kingdom; Web site www. yogaandhealthmag.co.uk/.

- *Yoga and Total Health:* A monthly magazine on practical matters. Get more information at www. theyogainstitute.org/magazine.htm.

- *Yoga + Joyful Living:* A quarterly magazine published by the International Himalayan Institute. Check it out at Yoga and Joyful Living, 630 Main St., Ste 300, Honesdale, PA 18431; Web site www. himalayaninstitute.org/yogaplus/.

- *Yoga Journal:* The most widely distributed (bimonthly) magazine on Yoga in the world. Find it at Yoga Journal, PO Box 51151, Boulder, CO 80322; Web site www.yogajournal.com/.

Seeing and Hearing All the Latest Audio Resources, DVDs, and Videotapes

Many Yoga teachers have produced their own DVDs and audio- and videotapes, of varying quality. Here we bring you a small selection of those tapes that we have listened to or watched and can recommend (including our own!). For a long list of available electronic resources, visit www. amazon.com.

Audio resources

- *The Lost Teachings of Yoga* by Georg Feuerstein
- *Yoga: A Basic Daily Routine* by John Schumacher
- *The Yoga Matrix: The Body As a Gateway to Freedom* by Richard Freeman
- *Yoga Nidra/Yoga Sleep* by Brenda Feuerstein
- *Yoga Wisdom* by Georg Feuerstein

DVDs and videotapes for Hatha Yoga and meditation

- *Gaiam Kids: Yogakids Fun Collection* by Gaiam
- *Kripalu Yoga/Dynamic* starring Stephen Cope
- *Kripalu Yoga Gentle* starring Sudha Carolyn Lundeen
- *Lilias! AM & PM Yoga Workouts for Seniors* starring Lilias Folan
- *Meditation for Beginners* starring Maritza

- *Relaxation & Breathing for Meditation* starring Rodney Yee

- *Total Yoga: Original* starring Ganga White and Tracey Rich

- *Total Yoga: The Flow Series — Water* by Ganga White and Tracey Rich (series also features *Earth* and *Fire* DVDs)

- *Yoga For Beginners* starring Barbara Benagh

- *Yoga For Families: Connect With Your Kids* starring Gerardo Diego

- *Yoga Journal: John Friend's Anusara Yoga Grand Gathering* (3 DVD Set) starring John Friend

- *Yoga for Stress Relief (with The Dalai Lama)* starring Barbara Benagh

General conditioning and Yoga therapy DVDs by coauthor Larry Payne

- *Classic Beginners' Yoga for Men and Women*

- *Common Lower Back Problems*

- *Common Upper Neck and Back Problems*

- *Immune Booster & General Conditioning, Levels One and Two*

- *Restorative Health for Women*

- *Weight Management for People with Curves*

Index

imbibation, 255–26
immune system, 530
India, 542–43
Indra Devi Foundation, 541
infant, 354
infertility, 343
inhalation
  breathing techniques, 130–45
  controlled breathing, 127, 144–51
  nasal breathing, 124–25
  yogic bends, 229
inner alertness, 470
inner ear, 195
insomnia, 110–13
Integral Yoga (style of Yoga), 54
Integrative Yoga Therapy organization, 537–38
integrity, 231, 453
intercostal muscle, 128, 182
internal oblique muscle, 205
International Association of Yoga Therapists, 484, 535
International Journal of Yoga Therapy, 550
International Yoga Studies program, 537
International Yoga Teachers Association, 541
intervertebral disc, 255
introductory class, 69
inversion exercise
  classic program formula, 332–33
  described, 215–16
  postpartum Yoga, 354–56
  props, 422, 427–28
  types of, 216–28
ischial tuberosity, 175, 253
ishvara-pranidhana, 454, 457–58
isometric movement, 138
isotonic movement, 138

Iyengar, B.K.S. (Yoga practitioner), 52, 423
Iyengar Yoga (style of Yoga), 52, 54, 275

J
Jacobs, Larry (Yoga practitioner), 423, 428
janushirshasana, 248–50
japa, 476
jathara parivritti
  described, 264–65
  variations, 262–63
  Yoga therapy, 505–7
jnana mudra, 166
Jnana Yoga (branch of Yoga), 45, 47, 546
Jois, K. Pattabhi (Yoga practitioner), 53
jumping frog posture, 365–66
junk food, 378

K
Kaivalyadhama Yoga Hospitalin Lonovola (organization), 484
kaki-mudra, 149
kapala-bhati, 150–51, 345
karate kid posture
  beginner's routine, 287–88
  described, 199–200
  older adults, 403–4
karma, 48
Karma Yoga (branch of Yoga), 45, 47–48, 546
karuna, 453
kidney, 233
Kinney, Shelly (Yoga therapist), 401
knee pain, 313, 319
knee-hugger posture, 372
kneeling sun salutation, 270–73
knee-to-chest posture
  classic program formula, 335

patience, 453

pause, during breathing, 135

perfect posture, 166–69

perfection, 86, 90, 527

perfume, 80

perimenopause, 388

periodical, 81, 549–50

Perry, Leroy R. (physician), 423

personal growth, 43, 531

Phoenix Rising Yoga Therapy program, 536

pigeon posture, 413–14

pillow, 421

PNF (Proprioceptive Neuromuscular Facilitation), 138

poise, 195

pollution, 123, 125

positive ion, 123

postpartum practice, 354–56

Postural Yoga (style of Yoga), 58

posture. *See also specific postures*

  adaptive postures, 94–95

  advanced practitioner versus beginner, 87–88

  balanced lifestyle, 64–65

  beginners' routine, 277–89

  benefits of, 156–57

  breathing techniques, 135–42

  defined, 49, 156

  described, 156–57

  foundation of, 171

  good habits, 525–26

  guidelines for practice, 90–94

  meditation tips, 469, 471–74

  number of, 86

  perfection, 86, 90

  purpose of, 156–58

  requirements, 90–91

Proprioceptive Neuromuscular Facilitation (PNF), 138
prostatitis, 217
psoas, 488
public class, 73–74
pure consciousness, 441
purity, 454
push-down exercise, 207–8, 493–94

R
Raja Yoga (branch of Yoga)
  books, 546
  defined, 46
  described, 48–50
Rama, Swami (Yoga practitioner), 442
Ramamani Iyengar Memorial Yoga Institute, 543
receptive/passive relaxation, 102
reclining posture, 300–6. *See also specific postures*
rectus abdominis, 205
reference book, 545
relaxation
  benefits of, 102–3
  books, 549
  children's Yoga, 373–74
  classic program formula, 338
  described, 61
  morning routine, 434
  postpartum Yoga, 355–56
  posture sequencing, 320–23
  prenatal Yoga, 354
  props, 427
  sun salutation benefits, 272–73
  Yoga therapy, 508, 518–20
relaxation response, 101
The Relaxation Response (Benson), 101

581